TABLE OF CONTENTS

G000141607

TABLES

FIGURES

CHARTS

Acknowledgments

This report was prepared by Eva Jarawan, Lead Health Specialist, and Christine Pena, Senior HD Economist (AFTH3), with the assistance of Karima Saleh (Consultant), Jean Rutabanzibwa-Ngaiza (Consultant), and Gabrielle Rooz (Consultant).

It is based on a review of several documents provided by the Eritrea Ministry of Health, international and national consultants, and partners in the country.

Maureen Lewis (HDNVP) and Salim Habayeb were the peer reviewers. Makhtar Diop, Country Director (AF5CO), Oey Astra Meesook, Sector Director (AFTHD), Mathew Verghis, Senior Economist (ECSPE), and Shiyan Chao, Senior Health Economist (AFTH1) provided comments on an earlier draft.

We would like to express our appreciation to H.E. Minister Meky, Minister of Health, officials of the Ministry of Health, zoba health teams, and external partners for their participation in preparing the report, and a special thanks to Dr. Nadia-Al-Alawi for her quick response to our many requests for information. We would like to acknowledge the excellent support provided by Ms. Nathalie J. Lopez-Diouf, Program Assistant (AFTH3) and Ms. Helen Tadesse, Program Assistant (AFTH1) in the processing of the report.

The views expressed in this paper are those of the authors and do not necessarily reflect those of the World Bank or officials of the Government of Eritrea.

Vice-President	Callisto E. Madavo
Country Director	Makhtar Diop
Sector Director	Oey Astra Meesook
Sector Manager	Dzingai Mutumbuka
Task Team Leader	Eva Jarawan

ACRONYMS AND ABBREVIATIONS

ARI	Acute Respiratory Infection
BoD	Burden of Disease
BOR	Bed Occupancy Rate
CHS	Community Health Services
CPR	Contraceptive Prevalence Rate
DOTS	Directly Observed Treatment Standards
EDHS	Eritrea Demographic and Health Survey
EHHSUES	Eritrea Household Health Status, Expenditure, and Utilization Survey
EPI	Expanded Program on Immunization
GOBI	Growth Monitoring, Oral Re-hydration, Breastfeeding, and Immunization
HMIS	Health Management Information Systems
IEC	Information, Education and Communication
IMR	Infant Mortality Rate
IMCI	Integrated Management of Childhood Illnesses
MCH	Mother and Child Health
MMR	Maternal Mortality Ratio
NRH	National Referral Hospital
PHC	Primary Health Care
TB	Tuberculosis
TFR	Total Fertility Rate
TT	Tetanus Toxoid
USAID	United States Agency for International Development
UNICEF	United Nations
WHO	World Health Organization
ZHS	Zoba Health Services

Currency Equivalent

Currency Unit = Nafka (NFA)
US$1 = NFA 10.1 (2000)

Fiscal Year

July 1–June 30

EXECUTIVE SUMMARY

I n March 2001, the Ministry of Health of the Government of Eritrea launched a process to
prepare a long-term Health Sector Policy and Strategic Plan (HSPSP) with a focus on assuring
equitable, quality, and sustainable health care. The Ministry of Health has outlined an open
participatory three-step process for developing the HSPSP, with active participation from all
partners involved in the health sector.

This Health Sector Note is the result of the first phase and serves as the preliminary basis for
further rounds of discussions and analyses among stakeholders to arrive at a strategic vision for the
national health sector.

This Note is a desk review based on available documents from various sources and of varying
quality and, as such, data comparisons should be viewed with caution.

Socioeconomic Situation

Of a total population of 4.1 million (2002), 62 percent are estimated to live in rural areas, a
decrease from 82 percent in 1995, and 38 percent[1] in urban areas, an increase from 27 percent for
the same period (EDHS 2002). Approximately 30 percent of the total population is comprised of
semi-nomadic, agro-pastoralists.

Eritrea remains one of the poorest countries in the world, with a gross national product per
capita of US$200 (1998). Approximately 60–70 percent of the population are classified as
living in poverty (1993–98), and unemployment rate in the non-farming sector is estimated at
15–20 percent. With respect to current employment status, 69 percent of men and 16 percent of
women aged 15 years and above were employed in 2002 (EDHS 2002). An overwhelming
majority (93 percent) of men in the workforce are in the 30–34 age group. Current employment
peaks at age 25–29 for women (26 percent).

---

1. The increase is primarily due to redefining some areas classified as rural in 1995.

There are no urban-rural differences by employment status for men, although employment rate among men is likely to be lower in the capital city of Asmara than in other areas. By contrast, women are three times as likely to be employed in urban than in rural areas.

The border conflict with Ethiopia, which started in 1998 and ended in 2000, has had a profound adverse effect on the economy—with the agriculture sector most affected, and the welfare of the population. Gross domestic product growth declined from about 8 percent in 1977 to less than 1 percent in 1999 (IMF 2001). GDP is estimated to have declined by 9 percent in 2000 because of an estimated 75 percent decline in crop production combined with the destruction and loss of physical capital.

An estimated 300,000 to one million people have been displaced during the conflict, representing 10–20 percent of the population, who now live under difficult conditions with inadequate shelter, sanitation, food and basic services. Approximately 90 percent of displaced households are headed by women. It is estimated that nearly 1.6 million people will require food and other humanitarian aid for another 12–18 months.

Lack of sustained economic growth does not hold much promise for a reduction in poverty in the short to medium term. This will constrain growth in personal income and government revenue, and in turn growth in domestic resources for investment in, and recurrent cost support to, the health sector.

Financial contribution from the population in subsistence agriculture for their utilization of health care services is likely to be minimal, if any. Increase in human capital, through literacy and other forms of education, will have to be matched by an increase in employment.

The Health Sector

Strengths

Since independence in 1991, the Government has made great strides in improving the living conditions of the population through expansion and rehabilitation of basic social infrastructure, such as health stations and schools. By 1999, 70 percent of the population were reported to have access to primary health care services (defined as being with 10 km of a health facility). In addition, most of the important public health programs, such as child health, expanded program on immunization, reproductive health program, nutrition, environmental health, information, education and communication, and community health services, are either being developed or under implementation.

The Government has made prevention and control of HIV/AIDS a national priority. MOH is working with other ministries, government institutions, NGOs, and external partners to curb the spread of HIV/AIDS, primarily through behavioral change.

MOH has initiated a new quality assurance program that includes technical efficiency and consumer satisfaction as two methods of assessing quality.

Increase in total MOH staff, such as physicians, nurses, health assistants, and sanitarians has been substantial. There are national schools for nurses and paramedics, although all physicians are educated outside Eritrea.

Several key activities related to pharmaceuticals are in the pipeline, including: a survey of traditional medicine practices; construction of three standard zonal drug warehouses; publication of the third edition of the Eritrean National List of Drugs and National Formulary; strengthening of drug quality control and introduction of new drug tests; inspection guidelines for drug manufacturing plants; disposal guidelines for expired and obsolete items; and improvement of logistics and the Health Management Information System.

Challenges

Despite the many positive developments outlined above, a number of challenges remain. Primary among them is the high burden of disease. About 71 percent of Eritrea's burden of disease is due to communicable and preventable diseases. Peri-natal and maternal health-related problems, as well as diarrhea and acute respiratory infection account for 50 percent of burden of disease share.

Public Health

Malaria is a major public health concern affecting 75 percent of the population. Yet, only 34 percent of Eritrea's households report having mosquito nets. Ownership of mosquito nets is higher in rural (37 percent) than in urban areas (29 percent).

HIV/AIDS has emerged as the leading cause of adult in-patient mortality and prevalence. Adult sero-prevalence rate is estimated to be 2.8 percent (UNAIDS/WHO 2001).

Tuberculosis was the second cause of in-patient case fatality in the age group of five years and above in 1998. Treatment is still not reaching adequate numbers of the infected, especially in vulnerable populations.

Although both the Infant Mortality Rate and under-5 mortality are below average for sub-Saharan Africa in 2002 (48 and 93 per 1,000 live births, respectively), there still remain tremendous challenges to bring down high malnutrition rates. During the same period, 40 percent of under-5 children were underweight, with 12 percent classified as severely underweight, 38 percent are stunted, with 16 percent suffering from severe stunting. Wasting affects 13 percent of children of the same age group, and an alarming 50 percent of them are anemic. Lastly, close to 74 percent of children with diarrhea disease are under three years of age (EDHS 2002). Less than 50 percent of breastfeeding children between 7–9 months receive complementary foods.

The above child health statistics suggest that efforts should focus on: (i) education on weaning diets; (ii) nutrition for under-2 children and pregnant women; (iii) providing child caretakers with health education on re-hydration; (iv) improving sanitation; and in the long-term, (v) increasing girls' education because of the positive influence of mothers' education on child health.

There has been a significant improvement in coverage of expanded program on immunization, with an estimated 76 percent of children aged 12–23 months fully immunized in 2002 (who have received up to measles vaccine). Only five percent remain unvaccinated, compared to 38 percent in 1995. However, targeted efforts are needed to ensure that immunization services reach all age groups of children, particularly in the poor and nomadic groups, and that children receive all the required vaccine doses.[2] More emphasis needs to be placed on the Growth Monitoring, Oral Re-hydration, Breastfeeding, and Immunization concept of primary health care.

Women Reproductive Health

Several risk factors contribute to Eritrea's high maternal mortality ratio (1,000 reported deaths per 100,000 live births) and morbidity. These risk factors include:

- Low age at first birth (21 years).
- Absent or inadequate prenatal care. Although the number of women receiving antenatal care from a health care professional increased from 49 percent in 1995 to 70 percent in 2002, women in urban areas tend to receive care from trained health staff by a greater proportion (91 percent) than those in rural areas (59 percent).
- Low immunization coverage: only 28 percent of pregnant and women of child-bearing age received full immunization of at least two doses of Tetanus Toxoid in 2000.
- Inadequate obstetric care: only 28 percent of deliveries are attended by skilled personnel, compared to 86 percent in Sudan, 61 percent in Egypt, and 38 percent in Uganda.
- Low maternal nutritional status.

---

2. There are high drop-out rates for second and especially third doses of DPT and Polio.

- Complications from the (traditional) practice of female genital cutting or circumcision.
- Education plays a large role in enabling women to access obstetric services. An estimated 88 percent of women with some secondary education were assisted by trained health personnel in 2002, compared to 36 percent with a primary education, and only 12 percent with no education.

With a population growth rate projected at less than three percent per annum, an estimated Total Fertility Rate of 4.8 (2002), and very low use of modern contraceptive methods—only seven percent of married women use contraceptive methods, Eritrea's population growth is expected to increase by 24 percent by 2010. This expected increase will put considerable pressure on health care services. The major health burden will be from children and women of child-bearing age, as this sub-group will remain at 60 percent of the total population.

In order to maintain continued improvements in maternal (and infant and child) health, focus should be placed on appropriate health care programs for women, with particular attention to the disadvantaged and vulnerable groups, such as the nomadic communities. Further assessment of this sub-group is needed to ascertain the extent of health inequity, especially among women and children.

Poor access to improved water and sanitation, particularly in rural areas, is an issue. In 2000, only 42 percent of rural dwellers and 63 percent in urban areas had access to safe water supplies. About one percent of the rural population had access to some form of sanitary facility, such as a pit latrine, compared to 66 percent in urban areas. The Ministry of Health seeks to increase sanitation coverage from one percent to 30 percent by year 2005. To achieve this objective, the Ministry of Health will need to work closely with the relevant sectors in the rural areas.

The current state of waste management systems is inadequate. At present, household and health care waste, both solid and liquid, are collected and disposed by the municipality in urban and semi-urban areas in the country. There seems to be no segregation at the generation and disposal sites of any type of medical waste. Household and health care solid waste are disposed on the same sites with inadequate waste site protection.

Human Resources and Infrastructure

The number of local doctors is insufficient. About 45 percent of physicians employed by the Ministry of Health in 1999 were expatriates.

Skills mix among health staff needs to be improved, in particular the high ratio of administrative to medical staff, low ratio of medical specialists, and shortage of staff with appropriate training in management.

Low salaries, lack of incentives and motivation for staff, as well as poor infrastructure and accommodation in rural areas, exacerbate the human resources problem.

The increase in number of hospitals, without sufficient attention to capacity and availability of human resources, requires *immediate* consideration. It is critical that future expansion of health infrastructure be guided by Eritrea's new Human Resources Development Policy.

The Ministry of Health has embarked on a hospital reform program to respond to the above issues. Assessments are also ongoing to contribute to the health facility rightsizing plan.

Public Health Expenditures

Public sector spending on health accounts is estimated at about 65 percent of all health spending for 1999, donor contribution at 27 percent, and household contribution at 8 percent (excluding the private sector).

Donor dependency is high: 53 percent of the 1999 drug budget was financed by external assistance, compared to 47 percent of Government share. The long-term effect of this high external dependency sustained drug supply needs to be assessed.

The Ministry of Health is embarking on new initiatives to improve revenue collection at health facilities. However, these new initiatives, and the corresponding changes, need to be closely monitored and evaluated to ensure not only a smooth transition and sustainability of the new system, but also to gauge their impact on the consumers, particularly the poor and vulnerable groups.

Private Sector Role

Little is known about private delivery of health care services, except that most private clinics are located in urban areas, and that the private sector is primarily involved in the procurement and distribution of drugs. In 2000, there were 259 retail drug outlets. Fewer than 20 percent of medical care seekers use private facilities as a source of care.

Given the shortage of human resources in the health sector and low level of public sector salaries, public medical personnel, for the most part physicians, also work in the private sector as a way to supplement their income. Coordination between the two sectors is necessary, however, to avoid the emergence of a two-tier health system, with the public sector providing the poor with mediocre quality services because of insufficient resources, and the private sector responding to the needs of the better-off segment of the population. The Ministry of Health is conscious of that risk and has embarked on a serious program to improve health care quality.

Health Sector Management

The local and regional health administration capacity needs to be reinforced to enhance effectiveness of the decentralization of financial and managerial functions.

Pharmaceuticals

At present, all drug and medical supplies are imported, although some local production is expected to start shortly, mainly for packaging.

Drug storage, space and distribution procedures, management systems, as well as transport for drug disbursement need to be improved.

Laboratory Services

Laboratory services need to be reinforced to support the Ministry's on-going efforts to improve and expand national health care services.

Health Management Information System

While there is relatively good data collection and analysis, feedback to service providers and program implementers is limited. Critical data for decision-making, in the form of national health accounts and unit cost information for facilities, are missing and/or inadequate. Information on private sector involvement is lacking. Further data collection and analysis are needed, for example population-based, to improve the policy-making process.

Special Situations

Two population groups require special attention: the large number of the population affected by the border conflict with Ethiopia and those living in nomadic communities.

Recommended Next Steps

Eritrea faces a number of challenges in the health sector to achieve many of the Millennium Development Goals. Given its commitment to eliminate poverty, the Government is willing to take appropriate actions to achieve the desired impact on the health status and general well-being of the population. To this end, adequate resources need to be mobilized and made available to health care services, as well as to other related sectors, such as water and sanitation. However, given competing demands on the country's limited resources, actions in all sectors need to be prioritized. In the health and health-related sectors, the following actions are recommended:

Short-Term Priorities

- Establish baseline information for many of the MDGs, together with realistic targets, towards which Government efforts may be directed.
- Evaluate the performance and cost effectiveness of specific health programs to better assess the health care needs of, and interventions for, target populations, especially the vulnerable groups.
- Estimate the *National Health Accounts* (NHA) to better assess the health sector's sources and uses of funds.
- Evaluate *alternative sources of revenues,* including user charges, as well as public and private insurance options to sustain the current health care system. Given the extent of poverty in the country, user fees might not be an optimal option. Prioritization of strategies and interventions, including minimizing the system's inefficiencies, could maximize use of limited available resources.
- Undertake a needs-based master plan of health care facilities and equipment to include the private sector.
- Explore ways to expand private sector involvement in the delivery of health care services.
- Develop a staff training and development plan for the Health Management Information System to strengthen the flow of information, identify program needs, and establish a monitoring, supervision and evaluation system.
- Health worker skills and training needs should be assessed, including training in proper epidemiological surveillance and reporting, as suggested by the high proportion of undiagnosed illnesses (27 percent) at public health facilities in 1999.
- National environmental policies and regulations need to incorporate a strategy for health care waste management. This strategy needs to be accompanied by a health care waste management plan that includes budget requirements, authorities in charge, identification of capacity needs, and a monitoring plan. In addition, partnerships between the public and private sectors as well as civil society are needed.

Medium-Term Priorities

- Undertake unit costing studies at select public hospitals and ambulatory care facilities to evaluate the public system's technical efficiency.
- Provide the framework for a comprehensive and coherent development of the health sector, with the respective role of the public sector, private providers and NGOs clearly defined.
- Explore the potential for hospital privatization.

Long-Term Priorities

- Develop financing options for universal coverage, such as a national health insurance, or a combination of public-private insurance mechanisms.
- Develop and implement modern incentive-based provider payment mechanisms.
- Promote private sector integration and develop a rational policy towards private sector development.
- At the facility level, improve case management quality, focusing on hospital hygiene, improving provider-patient relations, and integrating innovations in Information, Communications, and Technology (ICT) into service delivery.
- Increase financial and management autonomy of public health facilities.

CHAPTER 1

INTRODUCTION

Background

In March 2001, the Ministry of Health (MOH) of the Government of Eritrea launched a process to prepare a long-term health sector policy and strategic plan ((HSPSP), with a focus on assuring equitable, quality, and sustainable health care. MOH outlined an open participatory three-step process for developing the HPSP, with active participation from all partners in the health sector. A diagram of the three-step process, action plan and timetable is attached in Annex A.

Step 1 is the preparation of a health sector review carried out by the World Bank, based on existing documentation provided by the Government and other sources, notably the World Health Organization (WHO), the United Nations Children's Fund (UNICEF), the United States Agency for International Development (USAID), Demographic Health Surveys. *Step 2* consists of conducting an in-depth health sector analysis along five sub-sector working groups: PHC, hospital reform, pharmaceuticals, human resource development, health financing, leading to the preparation of a rationale for investments in the future development of the health sector in *Step 3*.

This paper, the Health Sector Note, is the result of Step 1 of the process outlined above. It serves as the preliminary basis for further rounds of discussions and analyses among stakeholders to arrive at a strategic vision for the Eritrea Health Sector. The Note incorporates comments received from MOH central agencies, Zoba (regional) health teams, external partners working in Eritrea, and the World Bank Eritrea Country Team.

Any attempt to arrive at a strategic vision of Eritrea's health sector requires first a common understanding of the current performance of the health system in terms of how well that system: (i) enhances the health status of the Eritrean population; (ii) protects the population financially against catastrophic illness costs; (iii) provides equitable access to high-quality health care services; (iv) performs efficiently at both the macro and micro levels; and (v) is financially sustainable, given the country's projected low economic growth and high demographic trends. To this end, it is necessary to analyze the health system from different angles:

- A description of the present demographic and epidemiological situation, expected changes expected over the next 20 years, and the resulting effects on the underlying needs and demands of the population.
- An analysis of the current socioeconomic conditions.
- An assessment of the current health system performance, including the policy context.
- An identification of areas of the health sector where further analysis is needed.

This paper is divided into five chapters. Chapter 2 describes the current and projected demographic and epidemiological conditions in Eritrea in terms of population, age and sex structure, fertility, mortality, morbidity, dependency ratios, and population growth rates. Chapter 3 describes the country's health system, its organization, infrastructure and human resources, and compares Eritrea's health outcomes, inputs, and expenditures with other countries. The chapter concludes with an analysis of the strengths and challenges of Eritrea's health sector. Chapter 4 suggests some further analyses/studies for Phase 2 in the development of the comprehensive health sector strategy. Chapter 5 presents the recommendations on priority "next steps" in the short, medium and long term.

It is important to note that this is a desk review based on available documents from various sources and of varying quality. For example, the current Health Management Information System (HMIS) became operational only in 1998, and comparison of data prior to 1998 with data from the current system should be viewed with caution. In addition, the HMIS is based on facility-level data, while other sources of information, such as the 2000 EPI Coverage Report, is community-based, leading to differences in sampling procedures and denominators. A Demographic Health Survey (EDHS) was conducted in Eritrea in 2002 as a follow-up to the first EDHS of 1995, and some of the preliminary results have been incorporated into this report.[3] Lastly, the Eritrea Household Health Status, Expenditure, and Utilization Survey (EHHSUES) was completed only recently, a delay caused by the country's two-year border conflict with Ethiopia, which started in 1998 and ended in 2000. Only two out six zones were surveyed in 1997. Its results will be incorporated in Phase 2 of the HSPSP.

Socioeconomic Situation

Despite being a relatively small country of about 124 thousand square kilometers, Eritrea has varying geographic and climatic zones, and its population of 4.1 million includes nine heterogeneous, ethno-cultural groups, each with its own language. Christianity and Islam are the two dominant religions, each claiming about 50 percent of the population as followers. The country is divided into three main physio-graphic regions, which have an influence on *physical access* to a variety of services: central highlands, western lowlands and eastern lowlands. It has six regions (zobas) and 58 sub-regions (sub-zobas). In 2002, about 62 percent of the population resided in the rural areas. Approximately 30 percent of the entire population is comprised of semi-nomadic, agro-pastoralists.

Eritrea is a relatively young country. Since independence in 1991, the Government has made great strides in supporting the development and improvement of the living conditions of the population, even in the face of a devastated social infrastructure and impoverished population, the result of the protracted war for independence. Basic social infrastructure, such as health stations and schools, were rehabilitated and expanded, leading to a concomitant increase in school participation rates and access to, and utilization rates of, health services.

---

3. According to the EDHS Preliminary Report (September 2002), final results are not expected to differ significantly.

However, the escalation in May 2000 of the border conflict with Ethiopia and the recurring drought have had a negative impact on the country's earlier economic achievements, with the agriculture sector the most affected of all sectors. Gross Domestic Product growth declined from about 8 percent in 1997 to less than 1 percent in 1999 (IMF 2001), only a year after the start of the conflict. GDP is estimated to have declined by 9 percent in 2000 because of a decline in crop production, estimated at 75 percent, and the destruction and loss of physical capital.

The country's border conflict with Ethiopia also had a devastating effect on the population, with lasting consequences to this day. An estimated 300,000 to a million people[4] (or 10–20 percent of the population) were displaced from their homes, and although many of them have returned since the end of the conflict, they suffer from inadequate shelter, sanitation, food and basic services. Although widespread famine and disease outbreaks did not occur, partly owing to Government efforts to provide food and other assistance, the situation could deteriorate. It is estimated that 1.6 million people will require food and other humanitarian aid for another 12–18 months (IMF 2001). A direct result of the prolonged conflict and consequent dislocation of the population has been an increase in the number of households headed by women. Forty-seven (47) percent of households are now estimated to be headed by women, compared to 31 percent in 1995 (EDHS), and 53 percent are headed by men. Of the displaced households, 90 percent are headed by women because of the conscription of all men, aged 18–40, during the border conflict. The number of households headed by women is greater in urban (53 percent) than in rural areas (43 percent).

In terms of *human capital*, 45 percent of Eritreans aged 6 and above are uneducated, with the majority being women (52 percent). The EDHS 2002 data indicate that of those in school, female participation decreases, the higher the level of education because of early marriages and withdrawal from school to assist with household chores, for example. The primary gross enrollment rate in 1999 was 57 percent, an increase from 52 percent in 1998 (48 for women and 59 for men). Secondary gross enrollment rate was 21 percent. However, net enrollment rates are significantly lower: 38 percent and 14 percent for primary and secondary levels, respectively.

Literacy among the adult population (15 years and above) was 48 percent in 1999 (60 percent for men and 34 percent for women). Among the youth (15–24 years), literacy rate was close to 70 percent.

Economic Growth and Structure of the Economy

Eritrea remains one of the poorest countries in the world. Its Gross National Product per capita is US$200 (1998) and its GNP PPP per capita is US$984 (2000). Its nominal GDP per capita is only about US$173 (estimates range from US$160-US$190). Agriculture accounted for only 19.2 percent of GDP in 1999, while the industrial sector and services sector accounted for 28.4 percent and 51.5 percent, respectively.

In real terms, average per capita income in 1999 was about the same as in 1995 (Donaldson 2000b; Lagerstedt 2000). Approximately 60–70 percent of the population are classified as living in poverty (1993–98).

Excluding people working in the traditional farming sector, current unemployment rate is estimated to be 15–20 percent. In 2002, only 15 percent of women aged 15 years and above were employed, compared to 69 percent of men. Employment peaks at ages 30–34 for men (93 percent are employed) and 25–29 for women (26 percent). There are no urban-rural differences for employment among men, but women in urban areas are three times as likely to be employed than in rural areas. With respect to child labor (ages 10–14), the majority of this age group attends school (70 percent for girls and 78 percent for boys), with only about five percent

---

4. Estimates vary depending on the source.

working (four percent boys and one percent girls). This contrasts sharply with 39 percent in the labor force in 1997.

Government Sector and Public Debt

The border conflict with Ethiopia has also exerted severe pressure on public finances. Government expenditures increased over 100 percent in real terms between 1993 and 1999. Capital expenditures ranged from 30 to 40 percent of total government expenditures during the same period.[5] However, public revenues did not keep pace with public expenditures. Total revenue as a percentage of GDP steadily declined, from 43.3 percent in 1997 to 34.4 percent in 2000. Tax revenues followed the same pattern, decreasing from 20.4 percent in 1997 to 17.6 percent in 2000. Personal income tax comprised 13 percent of total tax revenues in 1999 and 19 percent in 2000. Its share of GDP was 2.4 percent in 1999 and 3.4 percent in 2000 (IMF 2001).

The fiscal deficit (including grants) increased from 6 percent of GDP in 1997 to 59 percent in 1999, to decline to 36 percent in 2000. To cover the fiscal deficit, the Government has been borrowing from external sources, mainly from development loans. Because of the highly concessional terms of the external debt, debt service as a percent of export was estimated at only 9 percent in 1999. However, external resources were insufficient to cover the widening deficit, and domestic bank financing expanded rapidly. As a result, both domestic and external government debt increased sharply, from a combined 45 percent of GDP by the end of 1997 to an estimated 178 percent by the end of 2000. Current concern about the total level of public debt may be warranted, as debt service relative to export has increased to 27 percent in 2000.

The above profile of the economy and public finance suggests the following:

- Lack of sustained economic growth does not hold much promise for a reduction in poverty in Eritrea in the short to medium term,[6] constraining growth of personal income and government revenue, and in turn, growth of domestic resources for investment in, and recurrent cost support to, the health sector.
- Financial contribution from the population in subsistence agriculture for their consumption of health services is likely to be minimal, if any. While recent improvement in agricultural output since the end of the conflict with Ethiopia suggests that government measures to improve agricultural output may increase income, issues such as land reform and its impact on the poor must also be taken into consideration. Increase in human capital through literacy and other forms of education will have to be matched by an increase in employment.

The Government will need to maintain a careful balance between the country's pressing development needs and the burden of excessive debt servicing. This balance will affect the pace of development of the health sector.

---

5. Insufficient information was collected regarding the overall levels, capital, and recurrent cost support from external sources to determine if resources from the Government and donors are underfinancing public recurrent expenditures in general.

6. Natural resources exploitation may contribute to more rapid economic growth.

CHAPTER 2

DEMOGRAPHIC AND EPIDEMIOLOGICAL SITUATION

Demographic Trends

Eritrea's population was estimated at 4.1 million in 2000 (Table 2.1), with a projected annual growth rate of 2.83 percent. Population growth is expected to continue in the next 20 years due to its relatively high fertility rates. Total Fertility Rate (TFR) is estimated at 4.8 (EDHS 2002), although TFR remains higher in rural (5.7) than in urban (3.5) areas. By 2020, Eritrea's population is expected to increase by about 50 percent. Between 2015 and 2020, population growth rate is expected to decline to 1.9 percent, with a population growth of 6.2 million (Figure 2.1). Population under 15 years of age is expected to decline, from 43 percent of total population in 2000 to about 38 percent by 2020, although in absolute terms, this sub-group will increase from 1.9 to 2.3 million. The largest percentage increase will be seen among the adult population (15–60 years of age), from 50 percent in 2000 to 58 percent in 2020 (Figure 2.2).

By 2010, Eritrea's population is expected to have increased by 24 percent. The major health burden will be from children and women of child-bearing age, as this sub-group will remain at 63 percent of the total population. Thus, over the next 20 years, the country will be confronted by the dual burden of communicable diseases as well as non-communicable diseases and injuries.

The following is a summary of the demographic and epidemiological trends that will shape Eritrea's health system over the next two decades.

- With sustained Government's focus on health and population programs, a significant decline in fertility could be achieved. However, even with the continued decline in total fertility from 6.7 births per woman in 1990 to 4.8 in 2002, Eritrea will not reach replacement level fertility within the next twenty years, and population growth trend is expected to continue.
- Life expectancy remains low, although it is above that of sub-Saharan Africa's average by about two years (Figure 2.3). Life expectancy increased slightly from 48.8 years in 1990 to 50.4 years in 2000 (49 years for men and 52 years for women in 1998). By 2020, life expectancy in

TABLE 2.1: DEMOGRAPHIC INDICATORS ESTIMATED, 2000–2020

Demographic indicators	Estimated 2000*	Projected 2005	2010	2015	2020
Population (millions)	4.10	4.60	5.10	5.60	6.20
Population change since 2000 (%)		12	24	37	51
Population Growth Rate (%)					
Urban (%)					
Population by Age Groups					
No. of Children under-5	0.7	0.7	0.8	0.8	0.8
% of Total Population	18	16	15	14	13
No. of Youth under-15	1.9	2.1	2.2	2.3	2.3
% of Total Population	45	45	43	40	38
No. of Women of Childbearing Age (15–49)	0.9	1.1	1.2	1.4	1.6
% of Total Population	21.3	23	24	25	26
No. of Labor Force Participation (15–60)	2.1	2.3	2.7	3.1	3.6
% of Total Population	50	51	53	55	58
No. of Elderly above-60	0.2	0.2	0.3	0.3	0.3
% of Total Population	5	5	5	5	5
Dependency Ratio (%)					
Total (under 15 and over 60)	100	97	91	81	74
Youth only (under 15)	90	88	81	72	65
Elderly only (over 60)	10	10	9	9	9
Elderly as % of total dependents	10	10	10	11	12

Demographic indicators	2000–05	2005–10	2010–15	2015–20	2020–25
Population Growth Rate (%)	2.3	2.1	2.0	1.9	1.6
Life Expectancy at Birth (years)	50	51	54	57	58
- Male					
- Female					
Life Expectancy at 15 years (years)	42	42	44	47	48
- Male					
- Female					
Crude Birth Rate	37.0	34.1	31.6	28.9	25.8
Crude Death Rate	14.0	13.1	11.5	9.9	9.5
Total Fertility Rate	5.2	4.7	4.1	3.5	2.9

TABLE 2.1: DEMOGRAPHIC INDICATORS ESTIMATED, 2000–2020 (CONTINUED)

Demographic indicators	2000–05	2005–10	2010–15	2015–20	2020–25
Infant Mortality Rate per 1,000 live Births	61	57	52	47	43
- Male					
- Female					
Under-5 Mortality Rate per 1,000 live Births	94	87	78	68	63
- Male					
- Female					
Ratio of IMR/Under-5 Mortality	1	1	1	1	1
Maternal Mortality Ratio per 100,000 live Births	998 1,131 (estimated)[1]				

*According to MOH, the Ministry of Local Government has conducted a survey that estimates the 2000 population of Eritrea as 2.83 million. The methodology of that study is currently being reviewed in light of the 1995 EDHS estimate of 3.5 million and taking into account the population displacement during the conflict with Ethiopia. MOH is also using a population growth rate of 3 percent in its estimates. These differences will be considered in Phase 2 of the HSPDP.
Source: World Development Indicators 2001, World Bank, Washington, D.C., 2001.
1/ Hill, Kenneth, C. Abou Zahr, and T. Wardlaw. "Estimates of Maternal Mortality for 1995". In *Bulletin of the World Health Organization, 2001*, World Health Organization, Geneva.

Eritrea is projected to increase to 58 years overall. Figure 2.4 illustrates Eritrea's position *vis-à-vis* its neighboring countries with respect to life expectancy. While most other countries show a decline in life expectancy due to the rising toll in deaths related to HIV/AIDS, life expectancy at birth in Eritrea is expected to show positive growth. Figure 2.5 shows that in 1990 Eritrea had one of the highest gender differentials in life expectancy at birth compared to its neighboring countries. This gender differential has slightly declined over the past decade.

FIGURE 2.1: POPULATION PYRAMID FOR 2000 AND 2020 (IN '000)

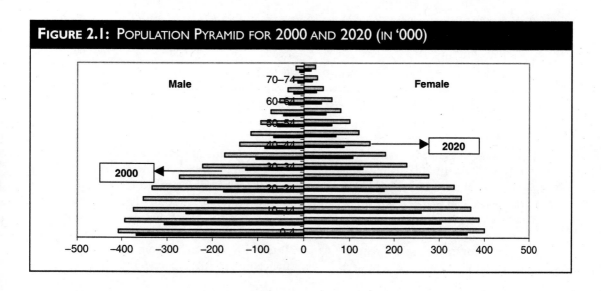

FIGURE 2.2: ERITREA, POPULATION PYRAMID FOR 2000 AND 2020 (PERCENT)

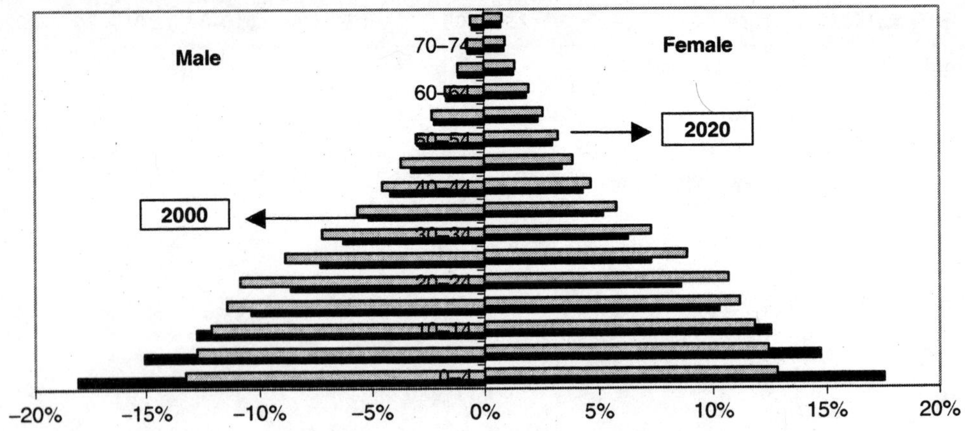

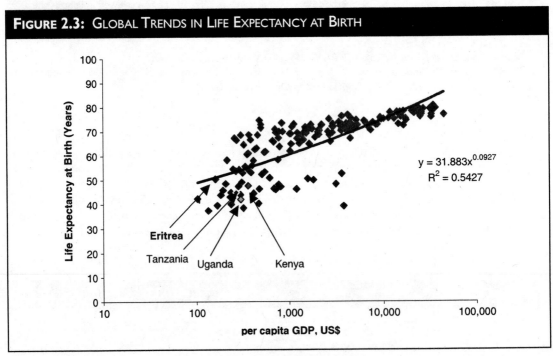

Source: *World Development Indicators* 2001, World Bank, Washington, D.C.

FIGURE 2.3: GLOBAL TRENDS IN LIFE EXPECTANCY AT BIRTH

$$y = 31.883x^{0.0927}$$
$$R^2 = 0.5427$$

Source: *World Development Indicators, 2001,* World Bank, Washington, D.C.

- ▤ Total age-dependency ratio remains high and has continued to rise during the past decade (Figure 2.6). In 2002, almost half of the population (EDHS 2002) was either under 15 years of age (43 percent) or above 65 (6 percent), resulting in a total dependency ratio of almost 100 percent, and an aged dependency ratio of 10 percent. The reduction in the total dependency ratio is expected to remain slow for the next twenty years, reaching 74 percent by 2020.
- ▤ Overall contraceptive use remains low in 2002, with no increase from the 8-percent level of 1995. However, the contraceptive prevalence rate (CPR) for modern methods has

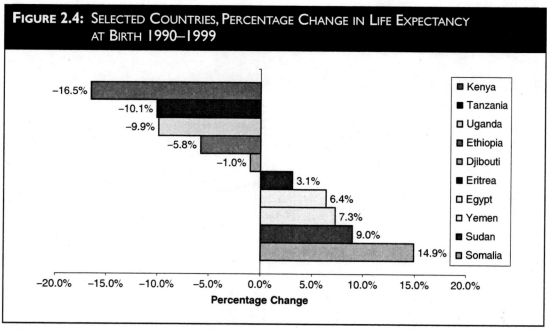

FIGURE 2.4: SELECTED COUNTRIES, PERCENTAGE CHANGE IN LIFE EXPECTANCY AT BIRTH 1990–1999

Source: *World Development Indicators,* World Bank, Washington, D.C., 2001.
Note: A negative sign indicates a reduction in life expectancy at birth between 1990 and 1999.

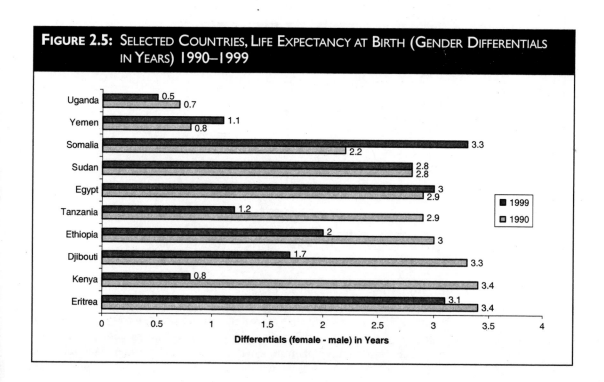

FIGURE 2.5: SELECTED COUNTRIES, LIFE EXPECTANCY AT BIRTH (GENDER DIFFERENTIALS IN YEARS) 1990–1999

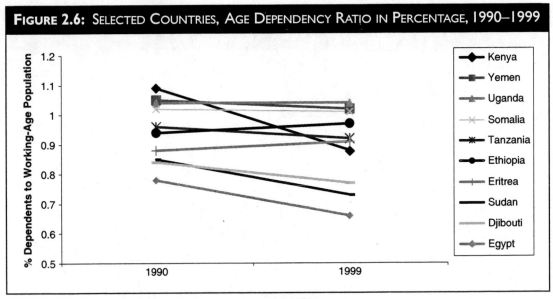

FIGURE 2.6: SELECTED COUNTRIES, AGE DEPENDENCY RATIO IN PERCENTAGE, 1990–1999

Source: *World Development Indicators,* World Bank, Washington, D.C., 2001.

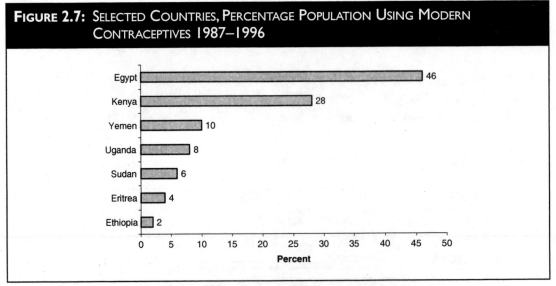

FIGURE 2.7: SELECTED COUNTRIES, PERCENTAGE POPULATION USING MODERN CONTRACEPTIVES 1987–1996

Source: UNFPA. *The State of World Population 2000,* (online) UNICEF Website, 2000.

increased slightly, from only 4 percent in 1999[7] to 7 percent in 2002.[8] As Figure 2.7 shows, CPR in Eritrea was one of the worst vis-à-vis its neighboring countries between 1987–1996. Recent DHS data indicate that a greater number of married women living in urban areas (17 percent), especially in the capital city of Asmara (23 percent), are more than four times as likely to use family planning methods than rural women (4 percent). Use of contraceptives is positively correlated with education. For example, 22 percent of

---

7. The 1995 EDHS reports CPR—currently married women who are using any method of family planning—at 8 percent, and for modern method at 4 percent.

8. This represents an increase from 50 percent of contraceptive users to 65 percent.

women with a secondary education or higher report using contraceptives, compared to 11 percent with a primary school education, and only 4 percent with no education.

Burden of Disease and Causes of Death

Eritrea still faces a high burden of disease (BoD) from communicable and preventable diseases. Around seventy-one (71) percent of BoD is due to communicable diseases (Figure 2.8). Perinatal and maternal health-related problems, as well as Diarrhea and Acute Respiratory Infection (ARI), constitute 50 percent of the BOD share. Most of these diseases are preventable. The high incidence of communicable diseases emphasizes the need for Eritrea to focus on preventive health programs and the provision of appropriate health care services to address communicable diseases and nutrition conditions. Highlights of the situation are provided below:

- In the above-5 population group, the top five causes of in-patient mortality in 2000 were consequences of Malaria, HIV/AIDS, TB, ARI, and Hypertension.
- According to facility-based reports, in 1998, TB was the second and HIV/AIDS the fifth causes of in-patient case fatality in this age group at the national level. In 1999, in just one year, HIV/AIDS emerged as the first major cause of in-patient case fatality for the same age group, to fall to second place in 2000 (MOH 2000a; MOH 2001b).
- Directly Observed Treatment Standards (DOTS) is estimated to cover 50–60 percent of the population. About 50 percent of diagnosed patients are smear-positive cases, most likely due to lack of diagnostic services. This should be at least 60 percent. The cure rate is reportedly above 60 percent (70–80 percent in Asmara), and lower in the rest of the DOTS areas. This cure rate is below standard and requires a detailed evaluation to determine the major problems and possible remedial actions.
- For adults aged 15–49, HIV-1 seroprevalence was 2.9 percent in 1999, with 49,000 adult cases of HIV infection (UNAIDS/ WHO 2001). The number of reported AIDS cases increased between 1996 and 1998, from 896 annual cases reported in 1996 to 1,610 cases in 1998.

FIGURE 2.8: PERCENTAGE SHARE OF BURDEN OF DISEASE, 1994

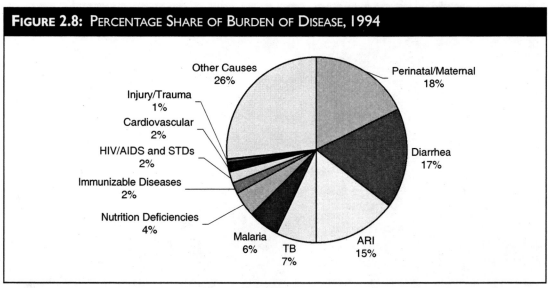

Source: Sebhatu, M., et. al., "Burden of Disease Study, Eritrea Summary Report". In *Proceedings of the East Africa Burden of Disease, Cost-Effectiveness of Health Care Interventions and Health Policy.* pp. 33–42. Regional Workshop, August 17–19, 1994. Asmara.

- Malaria is a major public health issue affecting about 75 percent of the population. Sixty seven percent of the population is at risk, especially under-5 children and pregnant women. Use of mosquito nets for prevention is low, as only 34 percent of households own mosquito nets. More households in rural (37 percent) than in urban areas (29 percent) own mosquito nets.
- Eritrea has a high coverage of iodized salt intake, with over 71 percent of households consuming iodized salts in 2002. Rural households were less likely to use iodized salts than urban households for reasons related to cost, poor distribution networks in areas with poor access to main roads, and local salt production.
- The high proportion of undiagnosed cases (27 percent) found in Government data for 1999 suggests the need to review health worker skills and training needs, including proper epidemiological surveillance and reporting.

Child Health

Eritrea's child health care indicators show poor health conditions among children. Diarrhoeal diseases are still a major cause of morbidity (and sometimes mortality) among the under-5. Yet, less than half who fall sick are taken to a health facility or are seen by a health professional. Malnutrition among children remains high, and as many as 50 percent of children are anemic. Special programs need to be introduced to combat poor child nutrition, and current program management needs to be strengthened to improve coverage efficiency and place more emphasis on the GOBI concept of PHC. With respect to immunization, EPI coverage has been extended, resulting in a substantial increase in full immunization for children aged 12–23 months, from 41 percent in 1995 to 76 percent in 2002:

- The Infant Mortality Rate (IMR) declined from 81 in 1990 to 61 in 2000 to 48 in 2002 (EDHS) and is below sub-Saharan African average (Figure 2.9). The under-5 or Child Mortality Rate (CMR) declined from 140 deaths per 1,000 live births in 1992 to 94 deaths per 1,000 live births in 2000 to 93 deaths per 1,000 live births in 2002. It is

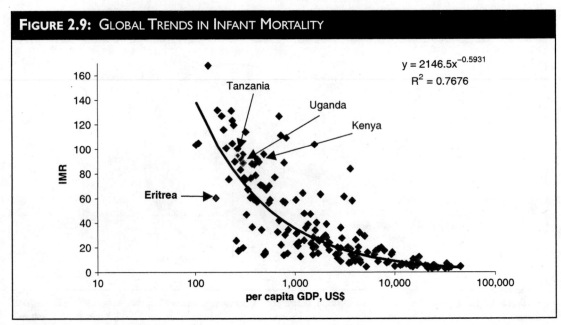

FIGURE 2.9: GLOBAL TRENDS IN INFANT MORTALITY

$y = 2146.5x^{-0.5931}$

$R^2 = 0.7676$

Tanzania

Uganda

Kenya

Eritrea

IMR

per capita GDP, US$

Source: World Development Indicators, World Bank, Washington, D.C., 2001.

also below the SSA average (Figure 2.11). Although decline in IMR in Eritrea shows steady progress, Government efforts to reduce infant mortality have been adversely affected by the conflict and the resultant population displacement. The disparities between rural and urban areas are reflected in the pronounced differences in IMR and rates for under-5 mortality. In 2002, the IMR was 48 for urban and 62 for rural areas. Under-5 mortality for urban areas stood at 86, while in rural areas the rate was 117. Under-5 mortality rates of over 100 were reported for four of the six zobas: Debubawi Keih Bahr (186), Semenawi Keih Bahr (154), Gash-Barka (123) and Debub (111).

▪ Under-5 child malnutrition is high, and there has been little change in the overall rates since the EDHS 1995. Thirty-eight (38) percent of children in this age group are stunted, and 16 percent are severely stunted (low height for age). Wasting (low weight for height) affects 13 percent , slightly down from 15 percent in 1995 (EDHS 1995). In 2002, 40 percent of Eritrean children were under-weight, compared to 44 percent in 1995–96 (WHO 2000a). Eritrea is one of the few countries where the proportion of under-weight children is higher than the proportion of stunted children (Figure 2.10).

▪ The prevalence of under-weight is usually high in the 6-to-24 month age group and is a reflection of low birth weight, poor nutrition in the early years, and low female literacy. The latest EDHS data confirms the pivotal role of girls' and women's education in improving child health. For example, stunting increases from 20 percent of children whose mothers are highly educated to 35 of children whose mothers have had primary level education, to 44 percent for children of uneducated mothers. These data emphasize the need not only for education on weaning diets and nutrition for children under-two and pregnant women, but also for increased access to education for women and girls. The EDHS 2002 found that less than 50 percent of breastfed children between 7–9 months received supplemental feeding other than breast milk. Sixty-seven (67) percent of

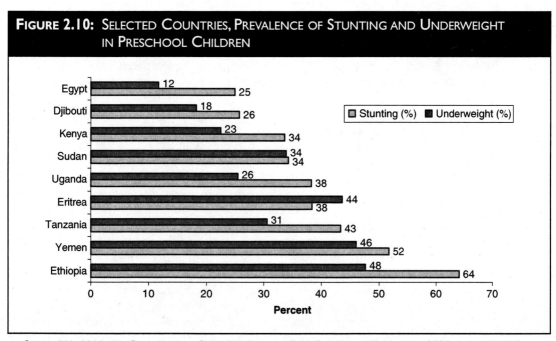

FIGURE 2.10: SELECTED COUNTRIES, PREVALENCE OF STUNTING AND UNDERWEIGHT IN PRESCHOOL CHILDREN

Source: World Health Organization. *Global Database on Child Growth and Malnutrition, 2000.* (online) WHO Website.

Note: Underweight is measured as children more than two standard deviations below the reference. median for weight-for-age; Stunting is measured as children more than two standard deviations below the reference median for height-for-age (Carlson and Wardlaw, 1990).

FIGURE 2.11: GLOBAL TRENDS IN UNDER-5 MORTALITY

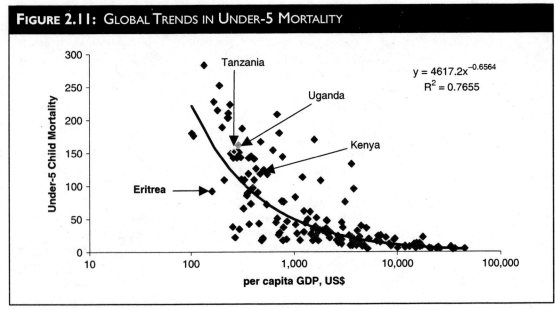

Source: World Development Indicators, World Bank, Washington, D.C., 2001

children under-four months are exclusively breastfed, which is similar to the DHS 1995 finding.[9]

■ Fifty percent of children under-5 suffer from anemia (associated with iron deficient diets and also malaria), compared to the regional average of 32 percent. Anemia is preventable, and Eritrea will need to focus on improving nutrition awareness and supplemental feeding programs.

■ Diarrhea prevalence for children under 3 was 24 percent in 1995. One in four children in this age group were reported to have diarrhea in the two weeks preceding the EDHS 1995, and about 66 percent of them received oral re-hydration therapy ORT (EDHS 1995). Although preliminary results from the EDHS 2002 discuss findings for the under-5 group (those reported to have had diarrhea in the two-week period before the survey), the data suggest a slight increase in the use of ORT by mothers (68 percent). Efforts need to be focused not only on providing health education on re-hydration, but also on actions to improve environmental health and hygiene, particularly in the rural areas and urban slums.

■ Nineteen (19) percent of children under 5 were reported with respiratory illness in the two weeks preceding the EDHS 2002, and 44 percent received some modern health care.

■ The top five causes of in-patient mortality reported in public hospitals and health centers in 2000 included acute respiratory infection (ARI); dehydration due to diarrhea, anemia and malnutrition; septicemia; and malaria.

■ With respect to morbidity patterns for under-5 children observed at public health facilities in 2000, cases of ARI comprised 40 percent of out-patient department visits, followed by diarrhea with 23.4 percent of cases. Others were eye and ear infections (7 percent), scabies and other skin infections (5.4 percent), malaria (4.3 percent), and anemia and malnutrition (2 percent).

■ According to routine reports from health facilities, immunization coverage for children under-1 improved from 1995–1999 (Table 2.2 and Figure 2.12), but declined to 43 percent in 2002, probably a result of the conflict. About 55 percent of children in this age group

---

9. The PHC division , MOH reported an increase to 98 percent exclusively breastfed children in 2000.

TABLE 2.2: IMMUNIZATION COVERAGE AND INCIDENCE OF IMMUNIZABLE DISEASES (1995–2000)

Immunization coverage and incidence of immunizable diseases	1995	1996	1997	1998	1999[a]	2000[b]	2000[c]	2002*
Immunization Coverage (%)								
BCG	44	52	67	71	64	61	90.1	91
Polio 3/DPT 3	35	46	60	60	56	52	85.5	83
Measles	29	38	53	52	55	50	81	84
Tetanus Toxoid (TT2+)	13	23	32	34	28	26.8	66	51**
Immunizable Disease Incidence								
(number of cases)								
Polio	10	0	41	—	—	—	—	NA
Diphtheria	0	0	—	—	—	—	—	NA
Tetanus—Total	1	0	0	3	21	—	—	NA
Tetanus—Neonatal	1	2	1	4	1	—	—	NA
Pertussis	125	45	—	119	132	—	—	NA
Measles	185	1783	777	316	320	—	—	NA

Source: [a] World Health Organization, Department of Vaccines and Biological. *WHO Vaccine Preventable Diseases: Monitoring System, 2000 Global Summary,* (online) WHO Website.
[b] MOH, Eritrea -2000 HMIS report.
[c] EPI Coverage Survey 2000, cited in MOH, *Eritrea Health Profile* 2000, May 2001.
* 2002 EDHS—Preliminary Report.
** Results are for women reporting at least one dose/shot of tetanus toxoid.

FIGURE 2.12: IMMUNIZATION COVERAGE FOR CHILDREN UNDER-1, IN PERCENT (1995–1999)

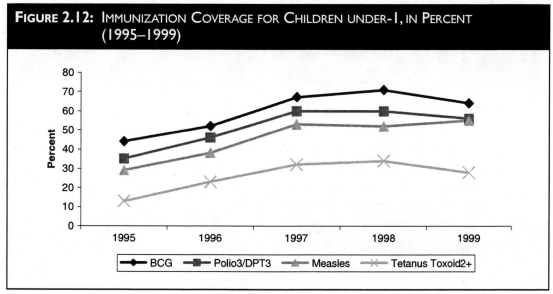

Source: World Health Organization, Department of Vaccines and Biological. *WHO Vaccine Preventable Diseases: Monitoring System, 2000 Global Summary,* (online) WHO Website.

were fully immunized (received up to measles vaccine) in 1999 (WHO 2000d). However, in 2002 (EDHS), the proportion of children fully immunized (12–23 months) was 76 percent, which is slightly lower than the 2000 EPI coverage survey showing a higher immunization rate of 79.4 percent. Differences in findings may be due to use of different denominators. Further analysis is needed to reconcile these differences.

- The incidence of immunizable diseases has been erratic. For example, 21 tetanus cases were reported in 1999, compared to an average of two cases between 1995 and 1998. Overall, the five-year trend shows a decline in most immunizable diseases among children under 1.

- Health facility reports show no case of Diphtheria since 1995 and no case of Polio since 1998.

- Thirteen (13) percent of newborns were low birth weight in 2000 (hospital data from PHC Division, 2000). At least 20 percent of BoD among children under 5 is attributable to conditions directly associated with poor maternal health, nutrition, and the quality of obstetric and newborn care.

Women's Reproductive Health

Eritrea has several of the risk factors for high maternal mortality and morbidity: relatively low age at first birth (about 21 years), absent or inadequate prenatal care, inadequate obstetrical care, high TFR, and low maternal nutritional status. Forty-one (41) percent of women had a body mass index (BMI) of less than 18.5 kg/m^2 in 1995 (EDHS 1995), indicating acute need for nutrition supplementation and education in the country. Complications of pregnancy and childbirth, most of which are easily preventable, are the leading causes of death and disability among women of reproductive age in developing countries. In order to maintain continued improvements in maternal (and infant and child) health, Government focus should be on appropriate health care programs for women. Some highlights are as follows:

- Antenatal coverage improved from only 49 percent of pregnant women in 1995 (UNICEF 2001a) to 70 percent in 2002 (Figure 2.13). Since 1995, antenatal coverage in rural areas and among uneducated women increased by at least 45 percent. Despite the substantial progress which must be acknowledged, urban-rural differences still persist,

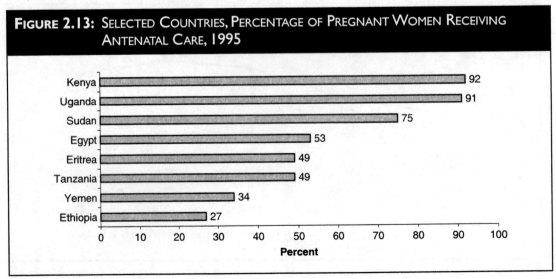

FIGURE 2.13: SELECTED COUNTRIES, PERCENTAGE OF PREGNANT WOMEN RECEIVING ANTENATAL CARE, 1995

Country	Percent
Kenya	92
Uganda	91
Sudan	75
Egypt	53
Eritrea	49
Tanzania	49
Yemen	34
Ethiopia	27

Source: UNICEF. *Global Database on Antenatal Care,* 2001, (online) UNICEF Website.

with 91 percent of women in urban areas receiving care from a trained health professional, compared to only 59 percent of rural women. In 1995, 85 percent of urban and
40 percent of rural women visited a modern provider for antenatal services. In 1999,
overall, about 40 percent of the target population of new pregnant women were registered in all health facilities (MOH, 2000a). This figure declined to 37.3 percent in
2000, although the 2000 EPI coverage survey reports a higher rate of 77.8 percent
(MOH, 2001b).

- Women's immunization coverage remains low. Twenty-eight (28) percent of pregnant and
women of child-bearing age received full immunization of at least two doses of Tetanus
Toxoid (TT) in 2000, a decrease from 34 percent in 1998 (health facility routine reports,
1998–2000). The 2000 EPI coverage survey indicates a higher figure of 66 percent.
Although the EDHS 2002 reports on women who have had at least a single dose of TT
(51 percent), the results may also indicate an increase in the number of women who
manage to receive two doses of TT. WHO recommends 90 percent coverage for three
doses of TT; for neo-natal tetanus to be eliminated, a high routine coverage of women of
child-bearing age, DPT for children and TT boosters.

- Between 1985–2000, deliveries attended by skilled health personnel were considerably
lower than in neighboring countries, except for Ethiopia (Figure 2.14). Only 21 percent
of deliveries received assistance from trained health professionals in 1995 (EDHS 1995),
increasing only slightly to almost 29 percent by 2000 (2000 EPI coverage survey). In
2002, 28 percent of all births occurring in the five years prior to the survey were attended
by a health professional; 26 percent of births occurred in a health facility compared to
17 percent in 1995. The proportion of rural women who deliver at a health facility is still
below 10 percent (from 7 percent in 1995 to 9 percent in 2002). In urban areas, the proportion of women who deliver at a health facility increased from 58 percent in 1995 to
62 percent in 2002.

- Women's average age at first birth was 21 years in 1995. Although this is above the average age for the sub-Saharan African countries (EDHS 1995), it is almost at borderline for
pregnancy-related risk.

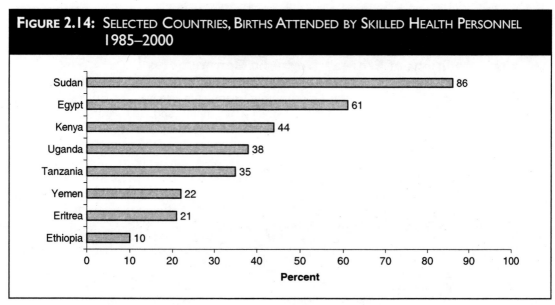

FIGURE 2.14: SELECTED COUNTRIES, BIRTHS ATTENDED BY SKILLED HEALTH PERSONNEL
1985–2000

Source: UNICEF. Global Database on Births Attended by Skilled Health Personnel, 2001, (online)
UNICEF Website.

FIGURE 2.15: GLOBAL TRENDS IN MATERNAL MORTALITY

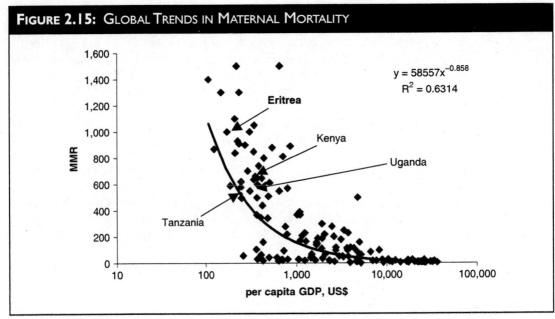

$$y = 58557x^{-0.858}$$
$$R^2 = 0.6314$$

Source: World Development Indicators, World Bank, Washington, D.C., 2001.

■ The Maternal Mortality[10] Ratio (MMR) is estimated to be well over 1,000 reported deaths per 100,000 live births (1993–98)[11]. Eritrea has one of the highest rates in sub-Saharan Africa (Figure 2.15).

■ Female genital cutting (commonly known as female circumcision) seems to be widespread, and its impact on women health needs to be assessed. Since the EDHS 1995, prevalence of female circumcision appears to have declined from 95 percent to 89 percent (EDHS 2002). The decline is notable among women under 25, indicating that some changes in practice are taking place. With respect to attitudes towards elimination or continuation of the practice, women were equally divided, with 49 percent for, and 49 percent against, continuation of female circumcision.

Health Conditions of Eritrea's Nomadic Communities[12]

About 30 percent of Eritreans are semi-nomadic or agro-pastoralists. Health conditions of women and children among the nomadic communities are below average for Eritrea. Among nomadic children, the most common health problems are anemia and ARI. Among women, immunization coverage is low, CPR is low, and abortion is common. Post-partum sepsis, bleeding and Cephalopelvic disproportion are common causes of mortality and morbidity during labor. Poor nutritional status and anemia are common occurrences among pregnant women. Maternal and infant mortality are above the country average. Malaria is endemic in the lowlands of Eritrea. Although Leishmaniasis is not endemic in Eritera, both cutaneous and visceral Leishmaniasis are prevalent in the low-lands and in some highland areas. Tuberculosis prevalence is high as well. Further assessment is required for this sub-population.

---

10. Maternal Mortality is usually defined as death occurring while the woman is pregnant or within forty-two days of termination of pregnancy, WHO.

11. MOH (2000a) reports a facility-based MMR of 240 per 100,000 births in 1999.

12. Data is taken from Tekeste, Tsehaye, and Dagnew (1999).

TABLE 2.3: MILLENNIUM DEVELOPMENT GOAL INDICATORS

Indicators	Current	Target (2015)
Poverty Rate (% of population below $1/day)	53[a]	20 or 22[b]
Net Primary Enrollment Rate (%)	33	100
Infant Mortality Rate (per 1,000 live births)	48	27 or 34[b]
Child Mortality Rate (per 1,000 live births)	93	48 or 52[b]
Ratio of Girls to Boys in Primary & Secondary Education	90 & 80	100
% Births Attended by Skilled Health Personnel	28	90
Use of Contraception—Any Method (Men)	NA	NA
Use of Contraception—Any Method (Women)	8	25
% of Population with Access to an Improved Water Source	7	25 or 75[b]

[a] Some estimates range from 60 to 70.
[b] Targets vary depending on the source.

Changing Epidemiological Profile

This previously isolated country is now open to trade, and Eritreans from the Diaspora as well as foreign investors travel in and out of the country. The armed border conflict of the past two years has displaced close to 10–25 percent[13] of the internal population, adding to the 200,000 returnees. The combination of varied geography, high mobility, and openness after isolation has contributed to the spread of communicable diseases and has complicated MOH's capacity to reach the population.

Eritrea and the Millennium Development Goals (MDGs)

As one of the poorest countries in the world, Eritrea faces a number of challenges with regard to achieving the MDGs. Table 2.3 summarizes Eritrea's current status and the MDGs by 2015. These indicators suggest that concerted and strategic efforts are needed in various sectors for Eritrea to successfully address poverty and enhance the well-being of its population.

With regard to *Infant Mortality and Child Mortality Rates,* one of MOH's major achievements under strengthening of the PHC programs is improved immunization services. Of children aged 12–23 months, 76 percent are fully immunized. Accessibility to immunization services within five kilometers has increased from 40 percent in 1995 to 97.4 percent in 2000 (MOH 2000). The Government has also adopted the Safe Motherhood and Integrated Management of Childhood Illnesses (IMCI) programs, which have also contributed to the reduction of IMR and CMR. IMR and CMR have improved since the EDHS 1995 results. In 1995, IMR and CMRs were 72/1000 and 136/1000, respectively, while 2002 rates are now 48/1000 and 93/1000, respectively. Whether the MDGs for IMR and CMR could be achieved may prove to be a challenging task. While decline in IMR has been significant in recent years, decline of CMR in Eritrea has been relatively slow, and the country has not made much progress relative to comparable countries because of local resource and staffing constraints.

To stem the high rates of *maternal mortality and morbidity,* MOH has adopted the safe motherhood program together with other complementary activities that include: increasing coverage of reproductive health services, adolescent health services and family planning services, as well as creating awareness on avoiding harmful traditional practices, such as FGM. More in-depth

13. Estimates vary depending on the source.

analysis is needed to ascertain whether the MDGs regarding *increases in percentage of births attended by health personnel and contraceptive prevalence* are realistic. At least three hospitals are presently under construction in Asmara, Barentu, and Mendefera, in addition to increased number of staff across all health facilities. Increases in the number of hospitals and health personnel are expected to have a positive impact on the availability of reproductive and maternal care services, especially for emergency care during delivery. Nonetheless, the expectation that the percentage of attended births would increase by almost 300 percent from 2000 to 2015 may be unrealistic, given the country's existing capacity.

A more detailed table of Eritrea's current status with regard to the MDG indicators for which data are available is in Annex G. The data gaps suggest an urgent need for baseline information on many of the MDG indicators and for the Government to confirm/establish actual targets towards which their efforts may be directed. *Completing the gaps in baseline information, establishing realistic targets, and agreeing on steps to attain them will be part of the second phase of the health sector strategy preparation.*

Complementary efforts are also needed in all other sectors. Establishing key priorities and targets is essential in the education sector to efficiently and effectively improve the skills and knowledge of the population. At the same time, improvements in infrastructure, business, and trade are also necessary to generate employment and productivity, and accelerate economic growth and development.

CHAPTER 3

ERITREA'S HEALTH SYSTEM

T his chapter describes the Eritrean health system. It is organized along the following
questions:

- What is the policy and governance context in which health care is delivered?
- What is the structure of the system in terms of public health care programs, delivery
  system including physical and human resources?
- How is the system financed?
- What methods are used to pay medical care providers?
- Given the demographic and epidemiological characteristics of the population, and the
  structure and financing of the system, what is the service utilization pattern?

As only limited data are available on the private sector and other public institutions involved
in health care provision (such as the military which has its own health care operations), this
chapter will mostly highlight the structure and delivery of the MOH.

Policy and Governance Context

After independence, the Government of Eritrea established a comprehensive macro-policy including strategies for food security, human resource development, with education and health as key
inputs, physical and social infrastructure development, and environmental restoration and protection. The Eritrean health policy supports the macro policy and aims to (a) minimize, and eventu-
ally eliminate, easily controlled diseases; and (b) enhance awareness of good health practices to
improve the productivity of the workforce. The main areas of focus of the health policy are:

- ensure the equitable distribution of health and social services to rural and urban areas, support primary health care, in particular improve and expand mother and child-care services;
- give special attention to major health hazards and promote health care services;

- encourage the private sector to actively participate in the provision of health services, following rules and regulations and operational modalities provided by MOH;
- promote community and beneficiary contribution in financing health services;
- introduce national health insurance schemes; and
- actively promote information dissemination on health practices (Tseggai 1998).

According to the Proclamation for the Establishment of Regional Administrations,[14] MOH role is to:

- formulate policies, prepare regulations, directives, standards, integrated plans and development of budgets, as well as supervise their implementation throughout the country;
- undertake research and studies, compile and collect statistical data;
- provide technical assistance and advice to regional programs and administration;
- comply with national policy, standards and regulations and, upon agreement of the Ministry of Local Government, assign regional executives, recruit, transfer, promote and dismiss employees; and
- seek external funding for regional development programs.

At the zoba[15] level, the main functions of the Zonal Medical Officers are:

- Planning, including the preparation of annual plans and budgets, project monitoring and, to limited extent, evaluation.
- Coordination of all development activities including those of the private sector and external agencies.
- Implementation—a core function at the zonal and sub-zonal levels. This involves managing relations with sub-regional and community administration officials, mobilization of community resources, handling contracts and financing mechanisms and providing support for operation and maintenance.

The Zonal Medical Officers report to both MOH and the Zonal Governor. For health sector matters, Zonal governors report directly to MOH. A detailed description of MOH (central and zonal levels) is in Annex C.

Planning and Budgeting

At the national level, Government coordination is through the Cabinet of Ministers. All funds are gathered through the revenue department of the Ministry of Finance and distributed through the Department of Treasury to the different line Ministries. No funds for health go directly from the National Government to the Zones. Funds flow from the Ministry of Finance to the Zones, but with the information also submitted to the line Ministry. Planning is consolidated at the national level. Salary payments and procurement have been decentralized to the Zones.

Planning for health—an exercise introduced three years ago—is made at the Zonal level (with contributions from lower levels down to the community[16]). These plans are consolidated and summarized at the national level. Similarly, the national level divisions and departments develop their own plans.

---

14. Government of Eritrea, Proclamation of Eritrean Laws No 86/1996: Establishment of Regional Administrations.
15. The zoba is the administrative division, corresponding to a region. Eritrea is divided into 6 zobas.
16. According to the Head of Zonal Affairs, Ministry of Health.

Budgeting is divided into capital and recurrent budgets, the former with a five-year perspective and the latter with an outlook for the coming three years. Recurrent budget estimates are based on historical figures. Once approved by the Ministry of Finance, the funds are made available to the zones on a monthly basis. Supplementary funds can be added each month at the request of the zones, upon approval by the Ministry of Finance. An internal audit is conducted each year.

Decentralization

The Government and MOH are committed to decentralization. In May 1996, the government adopted a policy to decentralize its operations, but implementation of the policy has been hampered by lack of skilled human resources at the zonal level. To date, fiscal decentralization has not been undertaken in the form of decentralizing budget expenditure decisions: whether government budget for health will be earmarked in general, and/or for specific programs; zonal governments cannot reallocate funds between sectors or retain revenues collected from health facilities.

Health System Structure, Coverage, and Capacity

MOH is responsible for public health, sector management and planning, health care delivery, and to a large extent, financing of health care for those who cannot afford it. In addition, Government regulates and controls the provision of private and NGO-operated health services.

Public Health

While the *Primary Health Care Policy and Policy Guidelines*[17] provide guidance regarding priority areas for programmatic intervention, the prescribed activities under this policy document are not supported by either cost estimates of providing these services, nor the cost-effectiveness of the strategies proposed. Health services in Eritrea are based on the principles of PHC and are made available to the entire population. They include promotive and preventive services, inter-sectoral activities, and community participation in health.

MOH is supporting several public health programs: child health; EPI; reproductive health program; nutrition, environmental health, and IEC; and community health services (CHS). Details about major public health programs are in Annex C. Limited information about the cost-effectiveness of some of the programs is in Annex E.

Health Care Delivery System

The public sector is the major provider of health care. Private clinics exist only in larger cities and serve a limited proportion of the population. At the village and district levels, the PHC network consists of health posts and health centers staffed with one or several nurses. Health centers have a laboratory and limited in-patient and delivery facilities. Many remote villages have no health facility. Every village or cluster of villages has teachers, extension and social workers, and malaria agents. They often work in cooperation with health facilities, sometimes referring patients. At the regional level, the recently established Zoba health team manages the PHC network. The Government is completing a network of referral hospitals (one in each Zoba).

Limited field observation (Lagerstedt 2000) show that the health system is in place and health facilities are well kept, clean and stocked with supplies, with the exception of the more remote facilities that need refurbishment and lack adequate staff, equipment, and supplies. MOH reports (2001b) also note overcrowding in referral hospitals and the *underutilization* of lower health facilities indicating possible quality issues, such as lack of adequate staff and services in these facilities. This issue needs further assessment.

---

17. MOH, September 1998.

Infrastructure

Health care services are delivered using a three-tier system:

- *Primary Level facilities* include *Health Stations*, the first contact for health services and the smallest health units, ideally serving a population of approximately 10,000. A registered nurse and one or two associate nurses staff the health stations. They provide mainly preventative care focusing on immunization, antenatal care, control and care of communicable diseases, health education and basic curative services. *Health Centers* are larger than Health Stations and serve populations of about 50,000. They have 25–30 beds and provide curative and preventative care, including polyclinic services, mother and child clinics, environmental sanitation, epidemic disease control and outreach services. Health Center staff may consist of two or three nurses, a laboratory technician, sanitarian, and a number of Associate Nurses, depending on the population of the catchments area. Staff at the health centers also supervise Health Stations and provide training to Community Health Agents and Traditional Birth Attendants.
- *Secondary Level facilities. First-contact or sub-zoba hospitals* serve populations of at least 50,000 and provide general medical and obstetric care and basic laboratory support services. Each hospital should have at least one general physician, a pharmacy technician, and several nurses, associate nurses, and laboratory technicians. They have facilities for minor surgical procedures and deliveries, and beds for in-patients. They are responsible for supervision of health centers in their locality. *Zoba referral hospitals* cater to populations of at least 200,000 and are typically located in zoba capitals. They provide general surgery, deliveries, laboratory, ophthalmic care, radiology, dental, obstetric, and gynecological services. They are also used as clinical training sites.
- *Tertiary Level facilities. National referral hospitals (NRH)* are specialized facilities located in Asmara and serve the entire country. These include: Halibet Hospital for medical and surgical cases for adults, Mekane Hiwot Pediatric Hospital, Physiotherapy Center, Behan Aini Ophthalmic Hospital, St. Mary's Psychiatric Hospital, Mekane Hiwot Obstetrics and Gynecology Hospital, and Hansenian Hospital, managed by an NGO.

MOH intends to re-categorize the above health facilities into the following: health stations, community hospitals (formerly health centers), regional hospitals, and national referral hospitals.

Expansion of Health Facilities

In 1993, Eritrea had about 16 hospitals, four health centers, and 106 health stations. MOH owned 46 percent of the total health facilities in the country. Since 1993, MOH embarked on PHC coverage expansion and decentralization policies that resulted in a significant increase of its share of health facilities. Between 1993–2000, 48 new health centers, 64 new health stations and 55 new clinics were constructed/upgraded. Table 3.1 and Figure 3.1 illustrates the growth in health infrastructure from 1990 to 2000. In 2000, MOH owned 88 percent of the total health facilities, and the remaining 12 percent were divided among the Catholic Mission (10 percent), the Evangelical Church (0.06 percent), and other NGOs (1 percent). The Catholic Church and other partners mostly own health centers, health stations and specialized clinics, such as MCH. Out of the seven hospitals in Asmara, *at least one is privately owned.*

Access to Health Facilities

Despite the increase in health facilities, and the vast improvement in coverage of the population for basic health care, access to facilities is still limited. For example, although MOH aims to have 10,000 people covered per health station, in 2000, on average, 24,000 persons were covered per health station. Health facilities are fairly well distributed across zones (Table 3.2), but there are high and low concentrations of health stations in some sub-zones (for example, there are places in Zoba Anseba where the distance to a health facility is more than 100 km).

TABLE 3.1: GROWTH OF HEALTH INFRASTRUCTURE, 1990–2000

Facility type	1990	1995	1999 Numbers	1999 Population per facility	2000* Numbers	Total growth (1990–2000) Numbers	Total growth (1990–2000) Percent
Hospital	16	16	18	222,000	18	2	13
Mini-hospital	0	4	5	798,000	5	5	1,200
Health center	4	40	49	81,000	52	48	60.3
Health station	106	130	154	26,000	170	64	
Clinics	0	31	37	108,000	55	37	
Total	**126**	**221**	**263**		**300**	**174**	**138**

Sources: Ministry of Health, *Annual Health Service Activity Report (January–December 1999)*, June 2000.
*2000 data from Ministry of Health Eritrea, *Eritrea Health Profile 2000*, 2001.

FIGURE 3.1: MOH HEALTH FACILITIES, 1990–2000

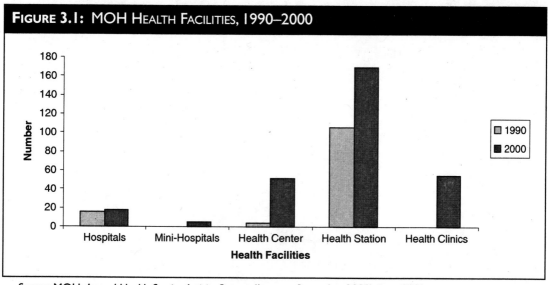

Source: MOH, *Annual Health Service Activity Report (January–December 2000)*, June 2001.

In 1991, only about 10 percent of the Eritrean population had access to a health facility within a 10-kilometer travel distance. With the growth in PHC facilities since independence, by 1998 approximately 70 percent of the population had access to a health facility within 10 kilometers. The EDHS 1995 provides information on the median distance of the survey respondents to service delivery points for EPI, FP, and MCH services. The median distance is between 7 and 9 kilometers. There is, however, wide regional variation in the accessibility to these basic health services. For example, the median distance to a facility providing delivery services by zones range from 2.5 km in the Central region to 20 kilometers in the Gash Barka region.

The Government has also developed a map illustrating the distribution of health facilities over the country (Annex D). This is an excellent tool to get an impression of the geographical distribution of health facilities in and between regions, but in a mountainous country like Eritrea, it needs to be interpreted with caution. Even though it may seem as if facilities are well

TABLE 3.2: DISTRIBUTION OF HEALTH FACILITIES BY TYPE AND ZONE, 2000

Facility	DKB	SKB	Anseba	Gash Barka	Debub	Maakel	NRH	Total
Hospital	1	4	1	3	3	0	7	19
Mini Hospital	1	0	0	0	2	1	0	4
Health center	3	11	8	12	10	8	0	52
Health station	14	24	23	38	45	26	0	170
Clinic	3	8	7	5	3	29	0	55
Pharmacies	0	3	2	2	2	22	0	31
Drug shops	4	1	2	1	2	18	0	28
Drug vendors	2	23	30	64	68	3	0	190

Source: MOH, *Annual Health Service Activity Report (January–December 2000),* June 2001.

FIGURE 3.2: GLOBAL TRENDS IN BED CAPACITY PER 1,000 POPULATION

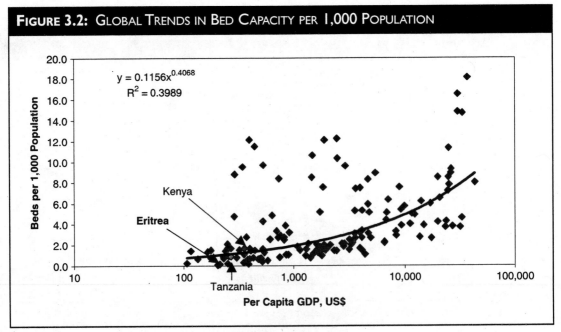

$y = 0.1156x^{0.4068}$
$R^2 = 0.3989$

Source: World Development Indicators, 2001, World Bank, Washington, D.C.

distributed, equity in terms of access may be difficult to achieve due to the non-availability of roads or the topography of the country.

Hospital Beds

A total of 3,126 hospital beds were reported for 2000, which translates into 0.76 beds/1,000 population. This is a small improvement from 1999, in which a total of 3,022 hospital beds were reported, or a 0.75 beds/1,000 persons (assuming a population of approximately 4 million). The total number of beds is expected to increase considerably, following the construction of new hospitals. Nevertheless, Eritrea's hospital bed-to-population ratio is below average for the sub-Saharan Africa region of 1.37 beds/1,000 persons (see Table F3, Annex F), and also below average for other countries worldwide with comparable income levels (figure 3.2).

TABLE 3.3: NUMBER OF BEDS AND BED OCCUPANCY RATE BY ZONES, 2000

Zones	Name of health facility	No. of beds	Bed occupancy rate
DKB	Tio	59	11.3
	Asseb	113	62.6
SKB	Massawa	187	22.6
	Ghinda	80	38.1
	Afabet	52	20.5
	Nakfa	93	26
Anseba	Keren	186	60.7
Debub	Senafe	42	29.4
	Dekemhare	60	N.A.
	Mendefera	102	32.2
	Adi Keyh	99	83.8
	Adi Quala	65	34.6
Gash Barka	Aqurdat	103	26.8
	Tesenei	84	44.3
	Barentu	41	52.9
Maakel	Edaga Hamus	54	36.3
National Referral	Mekane Hiwet Pediatric	200	52.9
	Mekane Hiwet Maternity	80	61.9
	Merhane Aynee Opthalmic	151	55.5
	St. Mary Psychiatric	170	129.2
	Hensennian	40	N.A.
	Halibet	336	80.5

Source: MOH, *Annual Health Service Activity Report (January–December 2000),* June 2001.

Bed Occupancy Rates (BOR) for 2000 range from only 11 percent in Tio Hospital to 129 percent in St. Mary's Pyschiatric Hospital in Asmara (Table 3.3). The optimal BOR is at least 80 percent but only three out of 22 hospitals had BORs above 80 percent: Saint Mary, Adi Keyh, and Halibet hospitals. BORs in zones are considerably lower than the National Referral Hospitals (NRH) and show wide variations. This could indicate a weak referral system, or patient preference to directly visit the NRH because of the perceived higher quality of care offered at these hospitals.

Human Resources
Between 1991–2000, the total number of staff in the MOH system increased from 387 to 4,906 persons, or by 1,168 percent (Figure 3.3). During that period, the number of physicians increased by almost 200 percent, from 58 to 173; only 44 percent were specialists. The number of nurses increased by 181 percent, from 288 to 811, while health assistants/sanitarians increased from 0 to 1,333. Administrative staff increased from 0 to 2,079 in the same period. Table 3.4 shows the development of human resources in MOH between 1991–2000.

Out of the total staff employed in 2000, 3 percent were physicians, 17 percent were nurses, and 27 percent were health assistants. Administrative staff represented 42 percent of MOH work

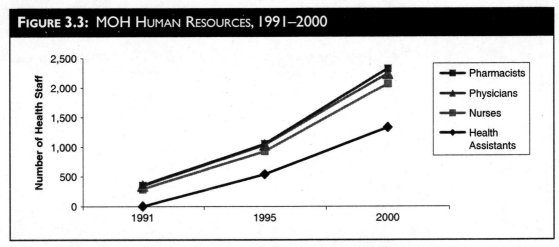

FIGURE 3.3: MOH HUMAN RESOURCES, 1991–2000

Source: MOH, *Annual Health Service Activity Report (January–December 1999)*, June 2000.

TABLE 3.4: GROWTH OF HUMAN RESOURCES IN THE MOH, 1991–2000

Category	1991	1995	1999	2000	Total Increase (1991–2000) Number	Percent
Physicians-GPs	58	108	100	100	42	72
Physicians-Specialist	0	0	45	73	73	
Nurses	288	391	735	811	523	181
Health Assistants	0	539	1,292	1,333	1,333	
Pharmacists, Technicians, Druggists	8	17	84	85	77	960
Sanitarians	0	15	21	21	21	
Lab Technicians	15	35	132	133	118	786
X-Ray Technicians	18	18	40	40	22	122
Other health professional staff	0	0	245	231	231	
Administrative Staff	0	1,425	1,790	2,079	2,079	
Total	**387**	**2,548**	**4,239**	**4,906**	**4,519**	**1,167**

Source: MOH, *Annual Health Service Activity Report (January–December 2000)*, May 2001.

force. The increase in the number of physicians and health assistants was mainly due to the return of professionals from exile overseas. The increase in the number of other categories was mainly due to continuous local training (MOH 2000a). Approximately 60 percent of MOH staff were women, mostly employed as nurses, health assistants, and custodial/manual staff. The distribution of private health professionals are not known at this time. Future inventories will include non-MOH, private, and NGO staff to give a more complete picture of all health professionals, although observations show that most private clinics may be staffed by public medical personnel, mostly physicians, working in their spare time to supplement their income.

FIGURE 3.4: GLOBAL TRENDS OF PHYSICIANS PER 1,000 POPULATION

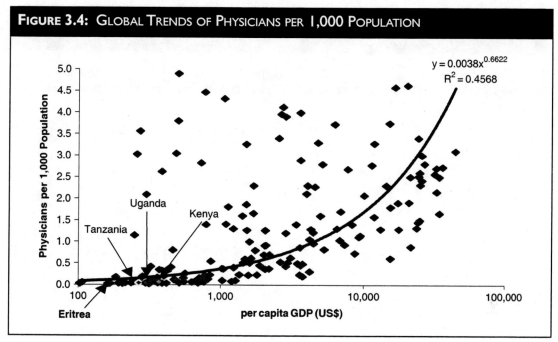

Source: World Development Indicators, World Bank, Washington, D.C., 2001.

Each physician covered a population of 23,033 persons, or 0.43 physicians per 10,000, and each nurse covered about 5,055 persons, or 1.97 nurses per 10,000 population. There were 4.5 nurses per physician and 7.5 health assistants per physician (or 1.6 health assistants per nurse) in the MOH system.

Eritrea's physician-to-population ratio is below average for the sub-Saharan Africa region, and also lies below the average for other countries worldwide with comparable income levels (Figure 3.4).

Even though the categories of health staff have increased each year, there are still acute shortages among some essential categories, especially internists, psychiatrists, ENT specialists, ophthalmologist, radiologist, and dentists. About 26 percent of the physicians employed by MOH in 2000 were expatriates from Russia, Sudan, Australia, China, Italy, the United States, and India.

Of the total health personnel in MOH, 42 percent are in the Center, with the remaining 58 percent distributed in the Zones. Maakel and the NRHs have the highest number of health personnel. Of the total staff, the following work in the NRHs: 46 percent are physicians, 36 percent are nurses, 19 percent are associate nurses, 22 percent are pharmacists and pharmacy technicians, 40 percent are x-ray technicians, and 26 percent are administrative staff. Taking into account only hospital staffing at the center and the zones, 68 percent of physicians, 68 percent of nurses, and 54 percent of associate nurses are assigned to the Maakel Mini hospital and the NRHs.

There is also a wide variation of health staff by Zone (Table 3.5). For example, in 2000 there were 8 physicians (GPs) in Maakel and 17 in Gash Barka. There were also hospitals without doctors (Tio Mini hospital, Afabet, and Nakfa hospitals) and midwives (Tio, Ghinda, Tesennei and Barentu).

Staffing norms per health facility are currently under development and review and were not readily available. However, local hospitals are expected to be staffed with a General Practitioner with training in minor surgery and competence to conduct a Caesarian Section, and equipped with laboratory services and x-rays. A Zonal hospital will have the four basic specialties (surgery, internal medicine, Obstetric and Gynecology and Pediatrics). The NRH will be the national

TABLE 3.5: DISTRIBUTION AND CATEGORY OF AVAILABLE HEALTH PERSONNEL PER ZONE, 2000

Category	DKB	SKB	Anseba	Gash Barka	Debub	Maakel	NRH	Unknown Residence	Total
General practitioner	9	11	11	17	15	8	27	2	100
Specialist	1	2	3	2	5	6	50	4	73
Nurse	29	52	55	76	98	141	292	68	811
Health Assistants	56	178	109	187	228	121	253	201	1,333
Pharmacist/ pharmacy technicians	5	7	9	7	12	26	19	0	85
Sanitarian	3	2	3	3	4	6	0	0	21
Lab technician	5	12	6	14	16	23	56	1	133
x-ray technician	2	5	4	6	6	1	16	0	40
Other health technicians	1	4	6	9	11	12	7	0	51
Other health professionals	2	15	13	32	17	51	44	6	180
Administrative staff	153	167	184	217	373	402	539	44	2,079
Total	**267**	**455**	**403**	**570**	**785**	**797**	**1,303**	**326**	**4,906**

Source: HMIS and Human Resource Inventory (R & HRD), cited in Ministry of Health, *Annual Health Service Activity Report (January–December 2000),* June 2001.

Note: Unknown Residence indicates that the current work place of some health personnel was not specified in their file.

medical center for the country[18]. Continued expansion of health facilities should take into account the need for all health facilities to have qualified staff and in sufficient number. In this regard, future developments must be guided by Eritrea's new Human Resources Development Policy.

Training of Health Professionals

Training activities are coordinated by the recently established Research and Human Resources Development Center in Asmara, which deals with training, continuing education, human resources planning, research, and Health Management Information System.

Most health professionals are trained at the Institute of Health Sciences in Asmara. The Institute includes the Asmara School of Nursing, the School of Medical Technology, Asmara School of Midwifery, and the Asmara Health Assistants School. Some are also trained at the University of Asmara, College of Health Sciences, which provides degree-level courses in nursing, pharmacy, and medical laboratory technology. However, *none of the medical doctors are trained in the country.* Between 1994 and 1999, about 54 percent of graduates from national institutions were females. Most trained professionals were employed by the Government after graduation.

For *pre-service training,* MOH recently merged and reorganized the five professional training schools (Asmara Nursing School, Asmara Health Assistant Training School, Midwifery School,

---

18. Discussion with Mr. Berhane Gebrintsae, Director General, Health Services Department (Lagerstedt 2000).

School of Medical Technology, and Gejeret School of Nursing) and upgraded them to a College of Nursing and Health Technologies (MOH 2001b). The purpose of this merger and upgrade was to standardize the quality of education and use resources more efficiently. Construction of a satellite campus for training of Associate Nurses in the College in Barentu is expected to start shortly.

As part of its *continuing education activities*, MOH has introduced a distance education program in collaboration with the University of South Africa. However, issues regarding limited information, communication, technology (ICT) capacity would need to be addressed before this program can be fully implemented.

In 1998, MOH conducted a comprehensive study to evaluate the training curriculum and presented the results in a workshop in December 1998. All curricula used to train health professionals were revised based on these results. It is important to assess how this training curriculum can be made more responsive and relevant to the needs of the population. The assessment could be done in line with the on-going preparation of the ten-year Human Resource Development Plan for Health and the review and ratification of the draft Human Resources Development Policy and Plan.

Pharmaceuticals

Procurement and Distribution

Eritrea relies on imports for all its pharmaceutical needs. Drugs and medical supplies are imported through PHARMECOR, a parastatal agency, and private firms. There are currently six importers and six wholesalers for drugs and/or medical supplies. Donated drugs are received in the Central Medical Stores and distributed to primary health care levels. The Department of Pharmaceutical Services within MOH is responsible for the control and distribution of drugs.

A new factory was expected to begin production and packaging of drugs in 1998 in Keren. The factory is nearly fully equipped but has not yet started production.

Private Sector Role

Private sector involvement in pharmaceuticals has been mainly through ownership of drug retail shops. In 2000, there were altogether 259 retail drug outlets, which included 31 pharmacies run by pharmacists, 32 drug shops run by pharmacy technicians, and 196 rural drug shops run by barefoot doctors, health assistants, and nurses. In 1996, 36 percent of PHARMECOR's drug expenditures were financed through the private sector. Total private sector expenditures for pharmaceuticals are not readily available, although according to MOH, they can be obtained from the importers themselves.

Financing

Public sector budget for pharmaceuticals was Nafka 35 million in 1999. MOH covered Nafka 16.6 million, or 47 percent of the total budget, and donors covered Nafka 18.4 million, or 53 percent. However, this budget was inadequate to cover the population's needs, and several in-kind donations of drugs were provided to the country by external partners. The Government has recently introduced a cost-sharing mechanism, through which patients pay for the drugs prescribed in the secondary and tertiary levels of health care. Evaluation is needed on cost-recovery through cost-sharing for drugs, as well as on government pricing and exemption policies, especially for the poor.

Current Status and Action Plan

The Department of Pharmaceuticals at the MOH has been actively strengthening institutional capacity and formulating drug procurement and distribution norms and standards. Since 1993, the following actions have taken place or are under review:

- Drafted the Eritrean National Drug Policy (1997), drafted and published the drug law, drug policy, standard list of drugs and treatment guidelines.
- Established Proclamation No. 36/1993 to control drugs, medical supplies and sanitary items.

- Developed Inspection Guidelines and Good Manufacturing Practice for private and public sector. Developed and distributed company registration guidelines, and Product Registration guidelines.
- Established the National Drug Quality Control Laboratory, introduced new drug tests, and developed standard laboratory operational procedures.
- Improved the distribution of retail pharmacy outlets, registration and licensing procedures of drugs and medical supplies importers; set requirements for licensing, and initiated licensing of wholesale importers;.
- Established and published the third edition of the Eritrean National List of Drugs in 2001. Published the Eritrean Standard Treatment Guidelines and drafted the Eritrean National Drug Formulary in 1998. The National List is generally well adhered to. In the public sector, more than 90 percent of drugs prescribed are from the list. Compliance with the list in the private sector is lower.
- For drug management, the following actions were taken: introduced—and established as a routine task—quantification of drugs and medical supplies requirements for the health facilities of the MOH; upgraded in 1998 computerized stock control system in the Central Medical Store; improved distribution efficiency and reduced the stock of expired drugs; and improved communication and reporting systems at both central and zonal levels; published in 1998 for the first time, Guidelines on rational storage and inventory control management for Central and Zonal Drug warehouses; computerized stock control system in the Central Medical stores in 1994 and upgraded in 1998,introduced computerization of stock control system at the zonal level in 1998; published guidelines on rational storage for lower health facilities in 1998; developed standard storage operative procedures; proposed design for the construction of 3 standard zonal drug warehouses.

The following key activities are in the pipeline: a survey of traditional medicine practices; construction of three standard zonal drug warehouses; publication of the third edition of Eritrean National List of Drugs and National Formulary; registration of products; strengthening of drug quality control and the introduction of new drug tests; inspection guidelines for drug manufacturing plants; disposal guidelines for expired and obsolete items; improvement of logistics and MIS; cabling of computerized stock control system at the central level, and upgrading of computerized stock management system at zonal level warehouses.

Laboratory Services
The national health laboratory structure of Eritrea is based on a three-tier system of peripheral, intermediate/regional, and central hospital laboratories, with the Central Health laboratory as the national reference. The Central Health Laboratory includes standardization of test methods, development of new technologies, implementation and monitoring of national quality control (include external proficiency testing) programs, in-service training of technical staff by conducting workshops and other forms of training. As a preliminary step towards quality accreditation, the laboratory participates in international external quality control programs.

While this has served the country's needs to date, it is insufficient to support the momentum of expanding national health services. Issues related to shortages in personnel, equipment and supplies; need for training and standardized internal quality control and preventive maintenance and repair; and lack of networking across different levels of health services facilities would need to be addressed.

An in-depth study of laboratory services in Eritrea will be undertaken shortly.

Health Sector Financing

Financing Sources
Overall, health care spending increased in nominal and real terms between 1995 and 1999 (see Annex E for details). Donor contribution increased in absolute terms and as a percent of total

health spending, from 20 percent in 1995 to approximately 30 percent between 1996 and 1999 (Donaldson 2000).

Total health care spending was estimated at 2 percent of GDP, with a public sector share of 55 percent (or 1.1 percent of GDP) and a private sector share of 45 percent (or 0.9 percent of GDP). Public sector contribution, as a percentage of GDP, increased to 2.9 percent in 1997, excluding all foreign assistance.[19] The current total health spending in Eritrea is not known.

Public sector spending on health is estimated at about 65 percent of total health spending for 1999, with donor contribution at 27 percent, and household contribution at 8 percent (excluding the private sector). Per capita health spending was estimated at Nafka 49. Detailed information on all private contributors, such as firms and private payments for drugs, as well as information on all public entities, such as the military and others, is unavailable. Exclusion or under-reporting of expenditures made by the Ministry of Local Government and donors is likely, as well as the value of in-kind donations of drugs. This issue will be addressed in Phase 2 of the Health Sector Strategy Options Preparation.

Trends In Public Health Capital And Recurrent Expenditures

- Eritrea's per capita GDP is below average of the sub-Saharan Africa region.
- Eritrea's per capita total health spending is not known, since private sector contribution to the health sector is not known.
- Eritrea's public health expenditure as a percentage of GDP is above average for sub-Saharan Africa region, and above average for other countries worldwide with comparable income levels (Figure 3.5).
- Eritrea's per capita public spending on health is below average for sub-Saharan Africa region, but close to the average for other countries worldwide with comparable income levels (Figure 3.6).

Total capital budget amounted to Nafka 24 million in 1999, representing an increase in real terms of 182 percent compared to the 1995 capital budget, but remained more or less constant in real terms between 1996 and 1999. Donor contribution remained high during the same period, and represented 63 percent of the total health sector capital budget in 1999, while Government contribution was 37 percent.

Total recurrent budget amounted to Nafka 133 million in 1999 and remained fairly constant in real terms for 1995–1999, with the exception of a sharp decline in 1996. Except in 1995 where a large portion of the recurrent budget financed back payment of ex-fighters, about 50 percent of the 1995–1999 recurrent budget was spent on salaries, 20 percent on drugs, and about 30 percent on other inputs, including operations and maintenance. Donor support increased from 7 percent in 1996 to 22 percent in 1999, mainly for pharmaceuticals. The country's dependency on external contribution for pharmaceuticals, and the long-term effects on maintaining constant drug delivery, needs to be assessed.

Since 1996, MOH revenues have increased in nominal and real terms, mainly due to an increase in registration and drug fees at health facilities. Revenues collected through such fees amounted to about 4 percent of the 1995 recurrent budget, and increased to an average of about 12 percent of the 1996–1999 recurrent budget. Historical details on revenues are not readily available. What is known is that in 1998–99, 80 percent of revenues came from registration,

---

19. The World Health Report (2000e) estimates Eritrea's total expenditure on health for 1997 to be 3.4 percent of GDP, of which 55.7 percent is public sector contribution, and 44.3 percent is private sector contribution, mainly in the form of out-of-pocket expenditures. Per capita health expenditure is estimated at US$6, and PPP US$24.

FIGURE 3.5: GLOBAL TRENDS IN PUBLIC HEALTH EXPENDITURE, AS PERCENT OF GDP

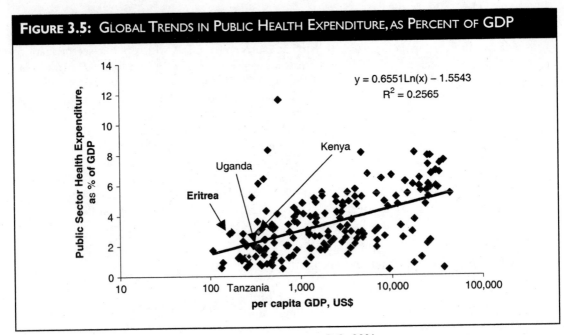

Source: World Development Indicators, World Bank, Washington, D.C., 2001.

FIGURE 3.6: GLOBAL TRENDS IN PER CAPITA PUBLIC HEALTH EXPENDITURE

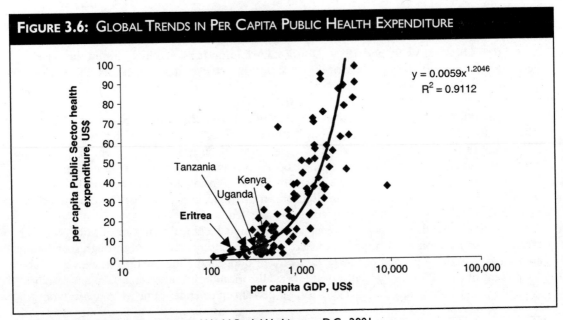

Source: World Development Indicators, World Bank, Washington, D.C., 2001.
Note: Only countries with a per capita Public Sector Health Expenditure of less than US$100 are shown here.

diagnostic, care and "hotel" services fees at MOH health facilities, and 20 percent were from drug fees.

Estimates of low, medium, and high scenarios of aggregate public health sector costs and financing from all sources (in real 2001 Nafka)[20] for the next five years indicate a financing gap between projected costs and available financing from public revenues and donor support for recurrent budget. The low scenario projects a shortfall of Nafka 58.1 million of a total budgeted cost of Nafka 204.7 million by 2007 (in real 2001 terms). The medium scenario projects a shortfall of Nafka 27.4 million of a total budgeted cost of Nafka 230.9 million. The high scenario projects a shortfall of Nafka 12.1 million of a total budgeted cost of Nafka 269.8 million.

Possible recommendations to address the above scenarios and bridge the financing gap include a careful assessment of: number of beds and other capacity needs, taking into account existing and planned infrastructure; intensifying efforts to identify additional donors for recurrent financing; and seeking ways to increase user fee revenue, with that increase being budgeted with the existing level of public financial support to the sector. However, given Eritrea's high rate of poverty, increases in user fees will need to be assessed carefully, especially in relation to PHC care, that is, how much can really be charged *vis-à-vis* how much people are willing to pay. Alternative strategies for health care financing will need to be identified to ensure universal coverage, especially for the poor. *Prioritization of interventions and minimization of inefficient use of resources would need to be carefully assessed during Phase 2 of the sector strategy preparation.*

Concerned with the financing of the health sector recurrent budget, especially in view of the large share of the public sector, MOH developed a health financing policy in 1996, which was updated in 1998. Implementation of the policy was however postponed because of the conflict with Ethiopia. By early 2002, MOH decided to reconsider its health financing policy and the roles and likely levels of financing from Government, donors, and the population using health services. In assessing the health financing policy, MOH needs to closely evaluate the proposed incentives to improve revenue collection at health facilities as well as the introduction of corresponding changes to ensure a smooth transition and sustainability of the new system. At the same time, efforts must be made to ensure that good quality health care is available to the poor and those unable to pay. The provision of good quality and affordable health care becomes particularly challenging because of the high poverty rate in Eritrea.

Household Health Care Utilization and Expenditures

Health Care Utilization

The Government does not regularly collect data on illness incidence, household health seeking behaviors, and household expenditures for health. Two household surveys were undertaken in the

---

20. The low scenario assumed a low rate of real GDP growth (1 percent), the medium scenario assumed a moderate rate of GDP growth (3 percent), and the high scenario assumed a high rate of growth (7 percent). Other key variables influencing health sector costs were rates of population growth and changes in the number of hospital beds. On the financing side, the same GDP assumptions applied to government budgetary resources for health, and increasing per capita levels of donor financing were assumed. User fee revenue was generally assumed to grow with GDP and population growth, but the "high" scenario assumed an ambitious target of collecting fees equivalent to 1 percent of GDP by 2010. The results of the "high" scenario should be regarded as the upper limit for the expansion of the costs and financing for the sector. Given historical rates of economic growth in sub-Saharan Africa, it is unclear that Eritrea will experience an average annual real rate of GDP growth of 7 percent. It is also difficult to predict trend in donor financing for health, and the real per capita level of donor financing may not remain constant considering population growth. Finally, while it is feasible that the population, on average, could pay 1 percent of GDP for health services, it is unlikely that the public sector will be able to mobilize this level of fee collection without altering access and quality of service (Donaldson 2002).

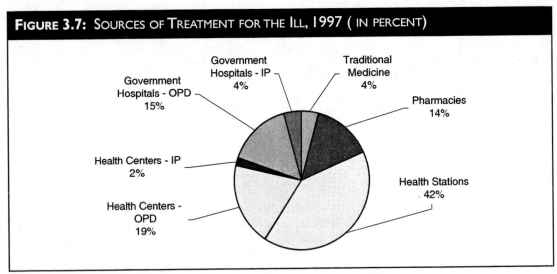

FIGURE 3.7: SOURCES OF TREATMENT FOR THE ILL, 1997 (IN PERCENT)

Source: Eritrea Household Health Status, Utilization and Expenditures Survey, 1997.
Note: Figures are rounded-off, and therefore may not add to 100 percent.

1990s. They are: the Living Standards Measurement Survey (LSMS) in 1996 for which results are not readily available, and the 1997 Eritrea Household Health Status, Utilization and Expenditure Survey (EHHSUES) conducted in the Debub and Gash-Barka zones[21]. Information in this section is mostly based on the EHHSUES.

The EHHSUES study found that most of those for whom illness was reported sought some health treatment. MOH health stations are an important source of health advice and service, with at least 40 percent of patients receiving care in those facilities. Private facilities were used as a source of care by fewer than 20 percent of medical care seekers (figure 3.7).

On the other hand, a 2001 MOH report underscores the major problem of overcrowding in referral hospitals and the underutilization of many lower-health facilities, because of understaffing in the lower level facilities and/or that "some services have not yet acquired a high level of acceptance in local communities" (MOH 2001d).

Health Care Expenditures and Methods of Payment

Fee for service is the most common payment method used for health care. However, health care fees are heavily subsidized by the Government at MOH health facilities. Health insurance is almost non-existent.

The EHHSUES shows that: (i) most patients pay for health care, even if a small amount; (ii) the majority of the population pay little for treatment aside from a registration fee and drugs; (iii) on average, households spend about 4 percent of their average monthly consumption (Nafka 11 per household per month) on health services; and (iv) of those households reporting illness, expenditure for health was about 6 percent of total household consumption (Nafka 28 per household per month, probably excluding travel and pharmaceutical costs). Compared to findings from other developing countries which show that poor households could be spending from 3 to 5 percent of their household consumption on health, consumption of poor Eritrean households on

---

21. Analysis of the data for the remaining four zones was not carried out due to the disruption of the conflict with Ethiopia. The preliminary draft report of the study in these two zones was based on interviews with 1,248 households, of which 686 (55 percent) indicated that they had a household member who was ill during the month prior to the survey.

health care may be higher. As MOH is embarking on new pricing and cost-recovery strategies, a closer look of its effects on consumers is required, particularly on the poor and vulnerable groups.[22]

In 1996, on average, 11 percent of MOH recurrent costs were recovered through user fees. In 1998, MOH developed a new Health Care Financing Policy, for which implementation was delayed because of the border conflict. The policy major objectives is to revise user charges for different categories of patients and review exemption scheme issues and cost assessments of different health care services as a basis for fee calculations. There is currently hardly any insurance scheme in Eritrea. The policy document also reviews the different areas of health insurance. It concludes that it would be difficult to implement an insurance scheme in Eritrea, partly because of low demand from, and equally low awareness of, the population of health care costs. However, application of the new fee schedule at MOH health facilities would increase annual government revenue from medical fees from the current level of Nafka 17 million to approximately an estimated Nafka 52 million, or by 206 percent.[23]

The Health Care Financing Policy needs to be assessed in light of current and projected health sector needs, together with estimated financing sources and the expected roles of the Government, external partners and the private sector, within the context of the country's high poverty rate, in order not to lead to a decrease in utilization of services by the poor.

---

22. Donaldson (2000) recommends that, based on current findings from Eritrea, the scope for increasing health fees be restricted to the higher income households in Eritrea.

23. This estimated amount is simply the current level of about 17 million, plus an additional 200 percent.

CHAPTER 4

PERFORMANCE OF THE HEALTH SYSTEM

This chapter summarizes some of the strengths and challenges in the Eritrean health care system that emerge from the previous analysis. It assesses the system in terms of how well that system performs in meeting the underlying health system goals of: improving health status, ensuring equity and access, promoting macroeconomic and microeconomic efficiency, assuring quality of care and consumer satisfaction, and being financially sustainable. Reform policies should build on the strengths while addressing the challenges facing the system. In addition, they will need to address the impending demographic and epidemiological changes facing the country.

Strengths

Health Programs

- The Government is committed to improving the health status of the population, as reflected in the macro and health policies, as well as in the Strategic Concerns. Program specific strategies and policy guidelines have been developed for all PHC components and for other areas. Government's commitment is also demonstrated by the increase in health care coverage since independence. In addition, most of the important public health programs are either being developed or implemented.
- The MOH is supportive of basic health care coverage and control of communicable diseases, as demonstrated for example by the active community participation and emphasis given to PHC in the health policy.
- Child immunizable disease incidence has decreased, and no cases of polio or diphtheria have been reported in the past few years.
- Tuberculosis treatment and policies are being developed, malaria vector control programs are being introduced, and iodine deficiency is being addressed through iodized salts.

MOH also considers the prevention and control of HIV/AIDS a priority. It is working with other ministries, government institutions, NGOs, and external partners to curb the spread of HIV/AIDS, primarily through behavioral change.

Health Systems

- Subsidized health care services are available at public health care facilities.
- MOH has initiated a new quality assurance program that includes technical efficiency and consumer satisfaction as two methods of assessing quality.
- The budgeting process and accounting system are in place with financial controls and auditing, although a performance-based budgeting process does not exist.
- The new HMIS is in place and is being followed by almost all local health facilities.
- Facilities of higher education exist for nurses and for paramedics. All physicians are, however, trained outside Eritrea.

Challenges
Public Health

- Despite existing PHC programs, communicable diseases remain high: perinatal and maternal health conditions, diarrhea among children and acute respiratory infections comprise 50 percent of the share of the burden of disease.
- HIV/AIDS has emerged as the second and first leading cause of in-patient mortality among adults in 2000 and 1999, respectively, compared to its position as the fifth cause of death in 1998.
- Availability of contraceptives is high, although utilization rates are low.
- Malnutrition and anemia among children and pregnant women continue to remain high.
- Immunization coverage, especially among women, needs to be further expanded.
- Maternal mortality is one of the highest in the region. According to the MOH 2000 Report, only 30 percent of women had met needs for health services in labor and delivery (including abortion).

Physical Access

- Poor access to improved water and sanitation, particularly in rural areas, is an issue.
- Poor access to health services for certain segments of the population, especially among the rural population and the nomadic communities, needs to be addressed.
- Although coverage has improved over time, there is still a wide variation between urban and rural areas. In addition, health service utilization continues to remain low for certain segments of the population, such as women and the nomadic communities. For example, few pregnant women avail of antenatal care services, and very few women deliver under the care of skilled health professionals. This issue needs to be further assessed, however, because poor utilization might be related to service quality issues. For example, MOH finds that hospitals are overcrowded while many lower-level health facilities are underutilized, partly because of understaffing in these facilities and perceived lower quality in services. Moreover, building more facilities might not necessarily be the right answer to the coverage problem. Different ways of service delivery, such as mobile services, might be needed.

Human Resources and Infrastructure

- The overall number of physicians and beds are low in comparison to the region and to the country's income level.

- The skills mix among health staff needs to be improved: there is a high ratio of administrative to medical staff, and low ratio of medical specialists.
- Shortage of managerial staff, or staff with appropriate training in management.
- Insufficient development of human resources. For example, job descriptions need to be updated and clear career growth tracks (including ranks and corresponding salaries) are not in place.
- Low salaries, lack of incentives and motivation for staff, as well as poor infrastructure and accommodation in rural areas.
- Increase in the number of hospitals, without proper attention to capacity and availability of human resources, needs *immediate* consideration.

Environmental Management

- The current state of waste management system is inadequate. Health care waste and contaminated health care waste handling, storage and disposal raise serious environmental and social concerns. At present, household and health care waste, both solid and liquid, are collected, transported and disposed by the municipality in urban and semi-urban areas in the country. It appears that there is no segregation at the generation and disposal sites of any types of medical waste. Household and health care solid waste are disposed on the same sites with inadequate waste site protection.

Financing

- The recurrent cost implications of the rapidly increasing number of hospitals needs to be urgently and carefully examined.
- Health spending overall, and public sector health spending, remain low by international standards, suggesting the need for Government to assess if it is adequately meeting the underlying health needs of the population. Increase in spending may not be possible, however, because of resource constraints. Significant increases in revenues from user fee increases may also not be realistic, given the country's high poverty rate. Ways to increase efficiency need to be explored, and priorities in interventions and services assessed and established.
- Most health facilities are reported to be experiencing a shortage of funds.
- Household health expenditure as percentage of their consumption may be high indicating the need to explore risk pooling/sharing mechanisms.
- There is no national health insurance.

Private Sector Role

- Little is known about private delivery of health services, except that most private clinics are located in the urban areas, and that the private sector is mainly involved in the procurement and distribution of drugs.
- Public medical employees may be practicing in the private sector as well as a way to supplement their salary.
- In the absence of coordination between the public and private sectors, there is a serious risk that a two-tier health system could emerge, with the public sector providing the poor with mediocre quality services because of insufficient resources, and the private sector responding to the needs of the better-off segment of the population. This could become increasingly apparent with costs associated with non-communicable diseases becoming more prevalent and more expensive to treat, particularly if public services are becoming increasingly budget-constrained.

Health Sector Management

■ It is likely that increased autonomy and professional management of public health facilities could increase the efficiency and quality of service delivery. Because health facility directors do not have full authority to manage the institutions, they lack the flexibility to adapt to changing local conditions and underlying needs of the population they serve.

■ Capacity will need to be built in local and regional health administration to enhance effectiveness of the decentralization of financial and managerial functions.

Pharmaceuticals

■ At present, all drugs and medical supplies are being imported, although some local production is expected to start shortly, mostly for packaging.

■ Eritrea relies considerably on external assistance for drugs and medical supplies and will need to explore avenues to lessen its dependency.

■ No information is readily available from MOH on private sector involvement and on the expenditures incurred by that sector.

■ Insufficient and inadequate drug storage space and distribution procedures and management systems, as well as transport for drug disbursement, need to be addressed.

■ Quality assurance issues will require focus and would need corresponding improvements in the amount and quality of trained personnel, facilities and equipment to ensure that quality improvement takes place.

Laboratory Services

■ Laboratory services are insufficient to support the ongoing efforts to improve and expand national health services. Issues related to shortages in personnel, equipment and supplies, need for training, and lack of standardized internal quality control and preventive maintenance and repair, as well as inadequate networking across different levels of health facilities need to be addressed.

The Health Management Information System

■ There is limited data analysis or feedback provided to service providers and program implementers. Critical data for decision-making, such as national health accounts and unit cost information for facilities, are missing and/or inadequate. Information on the private sector is lacking. Further data will be needed (some population-based) for policy making. There is potential to strengthen the HMIS.

Special Situations

■ The great number of the population affected by the border conflict, as well as those living in nomadic communities, require special attention. Destruction of health facilities, displacement of people, as well as mass repatriation of Eritreans living abroad combined with a large influx of refugees from Sudan, have added to the burden on the health care system. The impact of the recurring drought also needs to be assessed.

■ In collaboration with external partners and international and national NGOs, MOH has successfully managed the provision of health services despite these difficult circumstances. However, the management of physical and psychological trauma needs to be further assessed. According to MOH, between 1999 and 2000, the total number of reported cases of mental and behavioral disorder in hospitals and health centers has increased by 74 percent.

CHAPTER 5

RECOMMENDED NEXT STEPS

ny possible reform agenda should build on the strengths and address the challenges of the current health care system. Based on this very preliminary analysis of the health sector, the following priorities appear to emerge for the future. It is important to keep in mind that work on the medium- and long-term priorities should start in the near future for their implementation to take place in the next few years.

Short-term Priorities

- There is an urgent need for baseline information on many of the MDG indicators, and an equally urgent need for the Government to establish targets towards which its efforts may be directed.
- Given that 70 percent of the BoD are attributable to preventable, communicable diseases, there is an urgent need to focus on improving the provision and/or upscaling of preventive and other critical programs to address MCH, HIV/AIDS, sexually transmitted diseases, malaria and nutritional issues. In this regard, it is also important to evaluate the *performance and cost-effectiveness of specific health programs* to better assess the health care needs of, and interventions for, target populations, such as women, children, nomadic communities, and war-stricken population. Further population health care assessments might be required to direct resources to needy populations and improve critical programs.
- Estimate the *National Health Accounts* (NHA) to better assess health expenditures incurred in Eritrea. While rough estimates are provided in some reports for 1999, data available does not permit an analysis of patterns of health expenditures by health program, health facility, and geographical zone. Analysis of public expenditures, including donor resources, is a priority.
- Evaluate *alternative sources of revenues* including user charges, public and private insurance options, to sustain the current health system. Evaluate health care pricing, subsidies, user

charges, and fee exemption policies. Specifically, on the proposed user fee policy, carefully assess the following: what will the policy impact be on utilization of services, especially by the poor? what is the expected level of revenue? will local governments be able to support the costs of care for those to whom they issue indigency certificates? what mechanisms can be utilized for averting the problem of provider-induced demand for services? what will the impact of the proposed user fee policy be on the growth of the private sector and the distribution of health resources geographically? what are the recommended implementation guideline steps? *Note: work has recently started in developing a financial model that MOH can use for planning purposes.*

- Undertake a needs-based master plan of health facilities and equipment to include the private sector. This will help re-evaluate the public (and private) *investment strategy in the health sector*. A thorough analysis should be made of the *recurrent financing requirements of the sector*, based on current planned investment, and of the likely possible resources available to meet those requirements.
- Explore ways to expand private sector involvement, particularly privatization of hospital services.
- Undertake a study of the *management and organization of the health system* including the staffing and operations of MOH, other public and private entities, and the referral system. More specifically, to recommend:
  - *Human resource development* to: (i) finalize staffing patterns for different kinds of institutions and harmonize them with the services to be delivered in the system; (ii) compare the existing staff to the total staff needs based on staffing patterns of existing facilities, both public and private; and (iii) base training needs on the categories necessary to man the system, including private sector staff needs.
  - *Equity in Access* to: analyze the tier system in the country's public health system in relation to the services to be provided and in terms of levels of care; (ii) adapt existing facilities, over time, to this rationalized health system by down- or upgrading their function to the services needed for the catchment population; and (iii) analyze private facilities and their role in the future system in terms of what capacity they may have in the referral chain.
  - *Quality and Availability of Resources*: aiming to achieve quality does not begin at the point of services delivery. It begins with the design of the interventions to be implemented (design quality) and in ensuring that the quality and quantity of resources are matched with the design of the interventions. Thus, the four questions to be addressed are: (i) are planned interventions designed in such a way that they will ensure technical quality? (ii) are the resources allocated for the interventions sufficient, both in terms of quality and quantity, to achieve the quality aimed for? (iii) do patients perceive the services delivered to be appropriate to their needs? (iv) are the interventions implemented in such a way that expected technical quality is achieved?
  - Once decisions on what health care interventions are provided at each level of the referral system, define the drugs to be used at each level of care. Estimate and prioritize drug supply within the total resource envelope. This may lead to a revision of both the essential drug list and treatment guidelines.
- Explore alternatives, such as telemedicine, to address human resource constraints in service delivery, particularly with regard to the insufficient number of physicians.
- National environmental policies and regulations need to incorporate a strategy for health care waste management. This strategy needs to be accompanied by a health care waste management plan that includes budget requirements, authorities in charge, identification of capacity needs, and a monitoring plan. In addition, partnerships involving relevant stakeholders in the public and private sectors and civil society is needed.
- While the HMIS is one of the strengths of the Eritrean system, it continues to be a challenge, as there is a need to strengthen the flow of information, carry out an analysis to

identify program needs, and establish a monitoring, supervision and evaluation system. Operationalizing ways to improve the monitoring of data quality is important. Training is also very important because the availability of trained personnel has been identified as a major constraint in the further development of HMIS and the other components of Information, Communication, Technology in Eritrea (Ewan Technology 2001).

Medium-term Priorities

- Undertake unit costing studies in select public hospitals and ambulatory care facilities to evaluate the technical efficiency of the public system. Such information will serve as the basis for the development of efficiency-based provider payment systems.
- Provide the framework for a comprehensive and coherent development of the health sector, with the respective role of the public sector, private providers and NGOs clearly defined.
- Explore the potential for hospital privatization.

Long-term Priorities

- Develop financing options for universal coverage including: (i) a national health insurance system, (ii) financing some care through MOH, and (iii) financing care through a combination of public and private insurance mechanism.
- Develop, experiment, evaluate and implement modern incentive-based provider payment mechanisms including appropriate MIS and quality assurance systems to be used by all payers for purchasing both publicly and privately provided care.
- Promote private sector integration by providing incentives and through mechanisms such as certificate of need. Develop a rational policy towards private sector development.
- At the facility level, improve case management quality, focusing on hospital hygiene with patients; and integrate advancements/innovations made regarding Information, Communications, and Technology in service delivery.
- Increase autonomy of public health facilities to take financial and management decisions, including the revision of the statutes and staffing patterns at different levels of the health system.

ERITREA—MINISTRY OF HEALTH

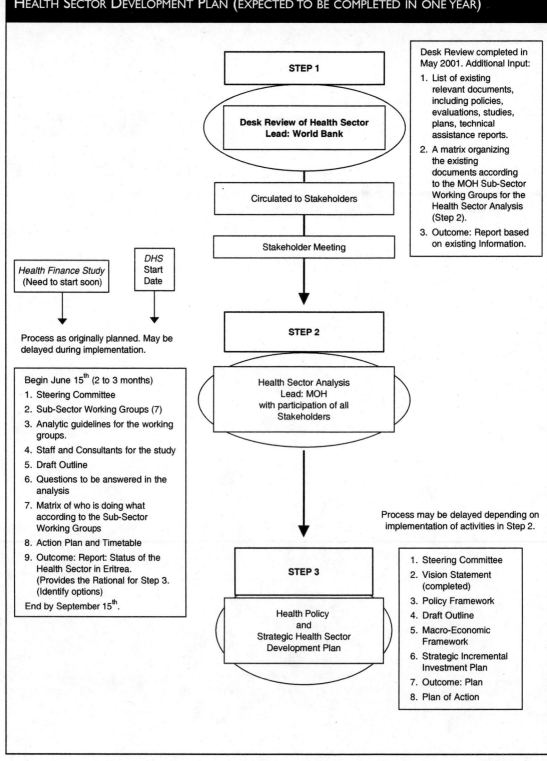

ORGANIZATION AND PROCESS FOR ESTABLISHING A HEALTH POLICY AND STRATEGIC HEALTH SECTOR DEVELOPMENT PLAN (EXPECTED TO BE COMPLETED IN ONE YEAR)

STEP 1

Desk Review of Health Sector
Lead: World Bank

Circulated to Stakeholders

Stakeholder Meeting

Desk Review completed in May 2001. Additional Input:

1. List of existing relevant documents, including policies, evaluations, studies, plans, technical assistance reports.

2. A matrix organizing the existing documents according to the MOH Sub-Sector Working Groups for the Health Sector Analysis (Step 2).

3. Outcome: Report based on existing Information.

Health Finance Study (Need to start soon)

DHS Start Date

Process as originally planned. May be delayed during implementation.

Begin June 15th (2 to 3 months)
1. Steering Committee
2. Sub-Sector Working Groups (7)
3. Analytic guidelines for the working groups.
4. Staff and Consultants for the study
5. Draft Outline
6. Questions to be answered in the analysis
7. Matrix of who is doing what according to the Sub-Sector Working Groups
8. Action Plan and Timetable
9. Outcome: Report: Status of the Health Sector in Eritrea.
   (Provides the Rational for Step 3.
   (Identify options)
End by September 15th.

STEP 2

Health Sector Analysis
Lead: MOH
with participation of all
Stakeholders

Process may be delayed depending on implementation of activities in Step 2.

STEP 3

Health Policy
and
Strategic Health Sector
Development Plan

1. Steering Committee
2. Vision Statement (completed)
3. Policy Framework
4. Draft Outline
5. Macro-Economic Framework
6. Strategic Incremental Investment Plan
7. Outcome: Plan
8. Plan of Action

ERITREA—TRENDS IN MACROECONOMIC INDICATORS, 1993–2000

Indicators	1993	1994	1995	1996	1997	1998	1999	2000
Population (millions)	3.39	3.48	3.57	3.67	3.77	3.86	3.96	4.07
% Below Poverty Line	69.0%							
% Employed			42.8%					
% Adult Literate						48.3%		
% Urban						18.0%		
GDP								
Nominal (million Nakfa)	2,866	3,730	4,031	4,538	4,713	5,028	5,828	7,098
Nominal/Capita (Nakfa)	845	1,072	1,129	1,237	1,252	1,301	1,470	1,745
Nominal/Capita (US$)				185	174	176	169	173
Real ('92 Nakfa)	2,628	3,294	3,136	3,397	3,467	3,172	3,395	
Real/Capita ('92 Nakfa)	775	947	878	926	921	821	857	
% Annual Change		22.1%	−7.2%	5.4%	−0.5%	−10.8%	4.3%	
% GDP								
Agriculture	17.8%	20.9%	17.7%	15.1%	14.5%		[a]17.1%	
Industry	3.7%	3.8%	3.6%	3.3%	3.1%		[a]29.2%	
Distribution	33.9%	31.8%	33.4%	33.7%	32.7%			
Other Services	19.7%	24.1%	23.2%	22.6%	23.0%		[b]53.7%	
Government Expenditures								
Nominal (million Nakfa)	1,415	1,602	2,703	2,557	2,532	3,832	4,629	4,944
Capital	455	430	572	839	1,119	1,496	1,984	1,643
Recurrent	861	1,018	1,672	1,523	1,402	2,337	2,644	3,301
% GDP	49.4%	42.9%	67.1%	56.3%	53.7%	76.2%	79.4%	69.7%
Real (1992 Nakfa)	1,298	1,415	2,103	1,914	1,863	2,418	2,697	
% Real Annual Change		9.0%	48.6%	−9.0%	−2.7%	29.8%	11.5%	
Government Revenue (million Nakfa)	893	1,027	1,521	1,420	2,044	1,751	1,700	2,101
Net Government Deficit	−522	−575	−1,182	−1,137	−488	−2,081	−2,929	−2,843
% of GDP	−18.2%	−15.4%	−29.3%	−25.1%	−10.4%	−41.4%	−50.3%	−40.1%
Public Debt (millions Nakfa)					1,758	3,263	5,601	7,595
Domestic (% GNP)					28.1%	47.3%	67.5%	67.2%
External (% GNP)					9.2%	17.6%	28.6%	39.8%
% GNP					37.3%	64.9%	96.1%	107.0%
Debt Service as % of Exports			0.4%	0.4%	1.0%	2.9%	9.3%	27.0%
CPI (1992 = 100)	109.04	113.24	128.56	133.58	135.93	158.49	171.65	
Exchange Rate (Nakfa/US$)				6.7	7.2	7.4	8.7	10.1

Source: Donaldson, Eritrea Technical Report, 2000.
[a] World Bank, *Eritrea At a Glance,* 2000.
[b] All services.

THE MINISTRY OF HEALTH ORGANIZATION STRUCTURE

CHART I: ORGANIZATIONAL STRUCTURE OF THE MINISTRY OF HEALTH

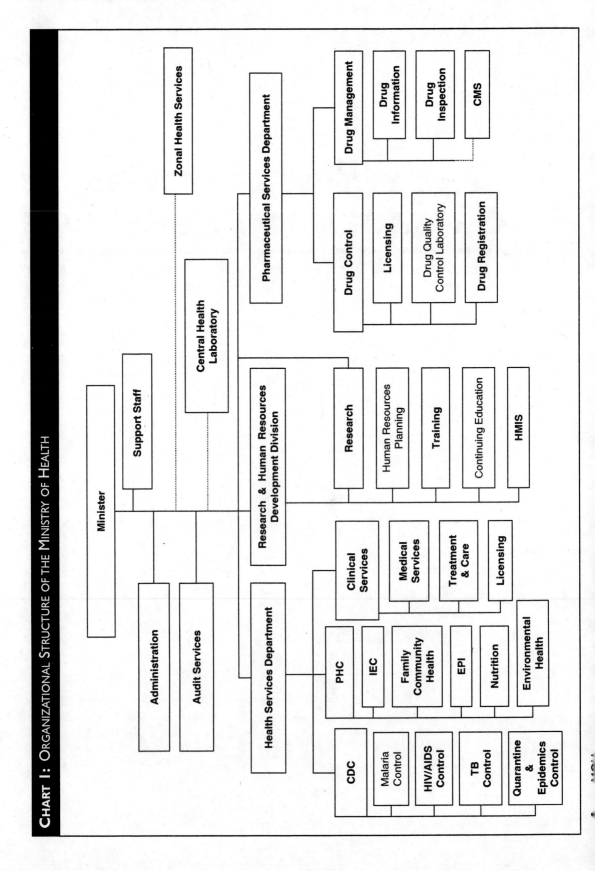

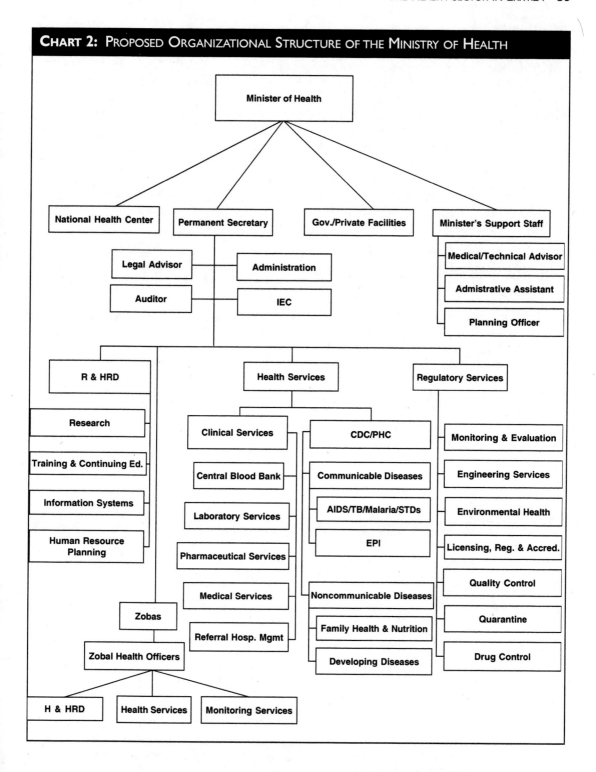

CHART 2: PROPOSED ORGANIZATIONAL STRUCTURE OF THE MINISTRY OF HEALTH

The Ministry of Health under the guidance of the Minister of Health manages the National Health System. Since the private sector and community health services are not fully developed, MOH is the principal provider of health services in Eritrea.

The Division of Administration and other support staff, together with the Offices of International Cooperation, Zonal Affairs Coordination and Public Relations assist the Minister in the Ministry's day to day operations. Personnel, Finance and Property and General Services and Maintenance are under Administration.

The Departments of Health Services (Primary Health Care, Communicable Disease Control, and Clinical Services), Pharmaceutical Services, the Division of Research and Human Resources Development, and Central Health Laboratory are directly accountable to the Minister.

The roles of the Ministry of Health are as follows, according to the Proclamation for the Establishment of Regional Administrations (Proclamation of Eritrea Laws No. 86/1996: Establishment of Regional Administrations):

- To formulate policies, prepare regulations, directives, standards, integrated plans and development budgets and supervise their implementation; throughout the country
- To undertake research and studies, compile and collect statistical data,
- To render technical assistance and advice to the regional administration
- Complying with national policy, standards, and regulations and upon the agreement of the Ministry of Local Government, shall assign regional executives and place the necessary facilities, recruit, promote and dismiss employees;
- Transfer of line ministry employees (with the knowledge of Ministry of Local Government)
- To conduct training, and render technical assistance for regional programs requiring professional input.
- To seek external funding for regional development programs.

The *organization structure for the zonal level* has the following outline:

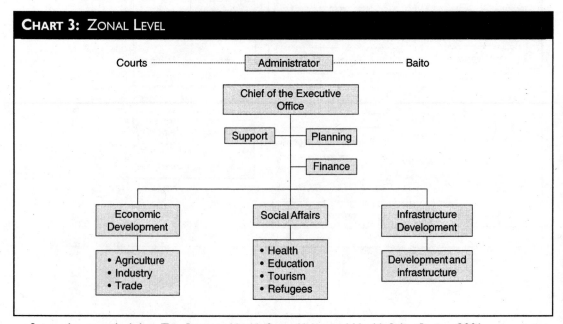

CHART 3: ZONAL LEVEL

Source: Lagerstedt, Adam. Trip Report, *Health Sector Vision and Health Policy Review,* 2001.

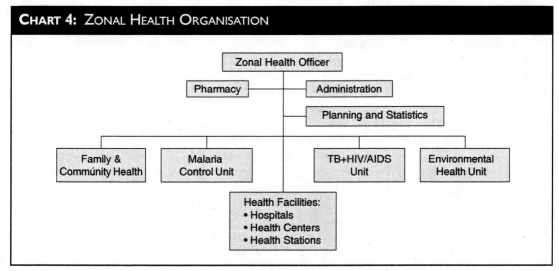

CHART 4: ZONAL HEALTH ORGANISATION

Source: Lagerstedt, Adam. Trip Report, *Health Sector Vision and Health Policy Review,* 2001.

The main functions of the Zonal level can be summarized as follows:

- *Planning:* this includes preparation of annual plans and budgets, project monitoring and to limited extent evaluation.
- *Coordination:* This mainly involves overall co-ordination of all development activities including private sector and external supporting actors as well as project beneficiaries.
- *Implementation:* This function appears to be the core function at the zonal and sub-zonal levels. It includes a wide range of tasks such as managing relations with sub-regional and community administration officials, mobilization of community resources, handling contracts and financing mechanisms and providing support for operation and maintenance.

The *organization for the health services* at the zonal level has the following outline:

The *Zoba Health Services* (ZHS) are part of the Department of Social Services of the Zoba. They are administratively accountable to the Zoba Administration which is directly under the Ministry of local Government. However, on technical matters, they are accountable to the Ministry of Health. The ZHS is headed by the Zonal Medical/Health Officer who leads the Zonal Health Management Team.

The Government has adopted decentralization as a national policy. Thus, MOH is in the process of establishing a decentralized health system in which the major portion of the duties performed at the central level will be executed at the zobas.

At present, the Zonal medical officer, together with his Health Team, plans for the activities of the Zone in an annually revised five-year plan, which is sent to the Ministry for evaluation and consolidation. Financing of the action plan is done through the Ministry of Health. The Zonal Governor cannot reallocate funds between different sectors.

Planning and Budgeting

At the National level, the Government is coordinated through the Cabinet of Ministers. All funds are gathered through the revenue department of the Ministry of Finance and distributed through the accounts department to the different line Ministries. No funds for health go directly from the National Government to the Zones.

Funds flow from the Ministry of Finance to the Zones, but with the information also submitted to the line ministry. Salaries are paid directly from the central Government to the staff employed. Planning is also consolidated at the national level. All procurement for the sector is also made centrally.

Planning for health is made at the Zonal level (with contributions from lower levels down to the community[24]). These plans are consolidated and summarized at the national level. The national level divisions and departments also develop their plans.

Planning at Zonal level was introduced four years ago and has been developed as an action/learning approach. No real guidelines exist, as the formats have been developed based on dialogue between participants in the planning process.

Budgeting is divided into capital and recurrent budgeting, the former with a five year perspective and the latter with an outlook for the coming three years. Even though each zone submits its own budget, these budgets are not compiled and submitted as the annual budget proposal for MOH. Rather, the recurrent budget estimates are based on historical figures. These estimates once approved by the Ministry of Finance is made available to the zones on a monthly basis. Supplementary funds can be added each month at the request of the zones upon approval by the MOF. An internal audit is conducted each year.

Main Strategic Concerns of the Ministry of Health

Equity in the distribution of health facilities, medicine, medical equipment, health workers and other public health activities under the PHC and CDC programs. This strategy aims to ensure universal access to available resources and services in order to provide coverage of the most important health needs of the population, with care provided according to need.

In majority of the cases, construction of health facilities is based on need as determined by population density and availability of health facilities and other factors including feasibility and status of being an administrative center. The number of new hospitals, health centers and health stations have increased by 92 percent, 58 percent, and 165 percent over the number of health facilities that existed before independence.

MOH estimates that access to health service (within 10 km radius or 2 hour walk) has improved from 46 percent in 1991 to 70 percent in 1999. More than half of the Eritrean population live within 5 km from a health facility.

Comprehensiveness of services so that preventive, promotive and curative health care measures can be provided in an integrated manner.

Appropriateness and cost-effectiveness of technology used and services provided. The kind and level of health facilities established, drugs and equipment used, and health professionals trained should be appropriate to the need and socioeconomic status of the country. For example, drug procurement is restricted to a list of essential drugs purchased through a competitive process. Also requires a shift from hospitals with costly specialist services toward peripheral levels of health system.

The Government does not accept assistance that does not adhere to its development policies and priorities.

Community Participation in identifying problems, prioritizing, planning and monitoring and evaluating programs/projects.

Promotion of inter-sectoral collaboration at the local levels in many aspects of primary health care. MOH recognizes health is closely related to other aspects of development and therefore there is a need to coordinate its actions with other sectors. Also communities tend to respond more readily to broad approach to development as opposed to fragmented sector by sector approach.

---

24. According to the Head of Zonal Affairs, Ministry of Health.

At present, at the zonal level, all social services and development programs are directly accountable to the local government—health, education, labor and human welfare are under one Director General in the local government which could facilitate a multi-sectoral approach to social services and development programs. Heads of various sectors in the zones are also members of the zonal council.

Though the structure of the local government is conducive to inter-sectoral coordination at the zonal and sub-zonal levels, capacity for effective coordination needs to be strengthened. There is also a need to clearly define the coordination mechanism at the central level. The HAMSET Control project has been cited in MOH documents as a good example of inter-sectoral collaboration.

Quality assurance so that performance standards are met. Since the initiation of the quality assurance program in 1998, the focus of quality assurance has expanded from concern with hospital patients to a concern for the total health system and from inspection/control activities by MOH to assigning responsibility to all health workers and the public. MOH has established a National Quality Assurance Committee (NQAC) as a focal point to facilitate quality assurance developments. A technical sub committee of the NQAC has been established to assist in daily work until a unit is established in MOH. Zonal quality assurance committees have also been established in all the zones. Facility based QA teams are also being established. Almost all high and mid-level managers from the center and zones and heads of most health facilities have attended at least a one week training course on QA. Development of policies and guidelines, clinical protocols, treatment guidelines and manuals are underway to establish national standards for quality and safety.

Human resource development. The major guiding principles of the HRD planning in MOH are: (a) establishing a national framework of training and development of health personnel, (b) optimal use of skills, experience, and expertise of all health personnel to ensure maximum coverage, cost effectiveness and quality of care; (c) minimize the mal-distribution of health personnel; (d) decrease imbalances among various types of health workers by ensuring the appropriate manpower mix; (e) Provide health workers with an appropriate career path through continuing education and different other training programs including in-service training, upgrading, distance learning, post-basic or specialized training; (f) establish a system of certification, registration and re-certification by assessing credentials and other methods by a certification and accreditation committee; (g) gradual decentralization of human resource management and administration including recruitment, deployment, promotion, etc, and (h) institutionalize regular performance appraisal and monitoring and using performance assessment/appraisal reports as the basis for staff career development and promotion.

To date, MOH has standardized and streamlined the different categories of health workers. It has also developed a standard training curriculum. The number of programs offered by the Institute of Health Sciences has increased from three (nursing, health assistance and midwifery) to ten to include laboratory and pharmacy technicians, physiotherapy and ophthalmic nursing, advance nursing, nursing, associate nurse, upgrading of associate nurses and medical technology.

MOH is also involved in developing curriculum and improving the standard of teaching in the Faculty of Health Sciences of Asmara University.

MOH is also making an effort to increase training opportunities through scholarships, fellowships and short courses abroad. It is also considering special admission criteria for candidates that come from the under-served communities who are willing to work for their community.

Health research. The overall objective of health research policy in Eritrea is to develop a national health research program, in general, and to provide policy guidelines for health research and direct research efforts to: address the priority health problems in the country, promote health and contribute to the socioeconomic development of the country, and enhance equity and social justice and promote a healthy society.

Main areas of concern have been identified; strategies have been drawn and some institutional capacity building measures such as building and equipping a central medical library. The Central

Health Laboratory has been rehabilitated, equipped and staffed for some basic research work in medicine and public health.

Health management information system. The objective of the National HMIS is to provide accurate, relevant, complete, and timely health information to support informed and appropriate health service, planning, and decision making at all levels of health care. Under the Research and Human Resource Division, a MIS unit was established. The National Automated HMIS was developed and started in all zones in 1998. Post installation support supervision were conducted in 1998 and 1999.

Among the recent additions to improve completeness of data are information on community health services, environmental health, military health, and necessary administrative activities.

Decentralization. The GOE and MOH state that they are committed to decentralization. Health services should be provided with the participation of decision-makers at different levels. MOH believes that strengthening of management capacity of zonal and sub-zonal level services is a precondition for effective decentralization. Decentralization should be accompanied by provision of resources and authority to the zonal, sub-zonal and health facility levels. At the same time, some health programs may benefit from a greater degree of centralized direction than others. MOH will seek to establish an appropriate balance between centralized guidance and local adaptation of policy to fit local realities.

Health financing. In 1996 and 1998, MOH was engaged in introducing and revising the system of user chargers for government provided health services. The 1998 health care financing policy seeks to provide improved guidelines to empower communities to share in the financing of health care costs. User charges will be part of a package of measures to improve service quality while maintaining accessible and affordable health services to those who cannot pay and ensuring that those who can pay do so. This necessitates a clear exemption policy. Public consultation and awareness creation regarding the fee increases are also necessary. In addition a mechanism must be established so that a proportion of collected funds is retained at the health facility level to finance service improvements. Local money handling arrangements need to be reviewed when fees are increased. The 1998 health care financing policy seeks to (a) upgrade the user's share of health care costs at secondary and tertiary levels and to replace the nominal fees by user fees at the primary levels; (b) achieve full cost recovery for clients who have health care coverage; and (c) grant exemptions for emergency cases for the first 24 hours, hazardous and contagious diseases, and people who are unable to pay and have indigence certificates.

In terms of measurable objectives, the 1998 HCF policy seeks to (a) increase health care cost recovery of recurrent costs by 40 percent; (b) improve health care efficiency, quality and equity by 50–60 percent; (c) decrease clients who pass the referral system by 60 percent so that they will be encouraged to use preventive health care services and discourage the use of expensive hospital care service for common and mild illnesses; and (d) increase community's participation in their own health care services by 70 percent.

Although health care financing reform was done in 1998, for a number of reasons which include the escalation of the border conflict, it has not yet been implemented and the 1996 policy is still being used.

Involvement of the private sector. MOH is encouraging private practice to be more effective and to ensure that it complements MOH services. It developed a policy on the Private Sector in 1995 and revised it in 1998. Individual practitioners who were given licenses to open "one-doctor" clinics were directed to change their mode of practice to provide comprehensive services with a number of physicians in the form of polyclinics. Practitioners are encouraged to get into contractual agreements with MOH to run state-owned institutions[25].

---

25. PHC division, MOH 5-year strategic plan, 2000.

Provision of drugs and medical equipment. One of the major responsibilities of MOH is to ensure the availability of safe and effective drugs of acceptable quality at a reasonable cost and the rational use of such products. The department of Pharmaceutical Services is the body entrusted to coordinate and supervise the implementation of the Eritrean National Drug Policy. As a regulatory arm of MOH, the Department of Pharmaceutical Services regulates all drug related issues based on existing regulatory system and policy. Structurally it has two divisions: Drug Control and Drug Management. The Department has five units: (i) Inspectorate Services, (ii) Quality Control Laboratory, (iii) Drug Information Services, (iv) Drug Registration and Evaluation, and (v) Licensing Unit. The immediate task of the Department is to develop a five-year action plan that outlines the approaches and activities in detail, including the budget and establishment of an advisory council and expert committees. The extent to which objectives are being met will be monitored and evaluated periodically.

Overview of Public Health Programs

A. Primary Health Care

Health services in Eritrea are based on the principles of Primary Health Care and aim at making PHC services available to the entire population. It includes promotive and preventive services, inter-sectoral activities, and community participation in health. The major public health programs are as follows:

Child Health. The overall objectives of the Integrated Management of Childhood Illness (IMCI) program are: (a) to improve the quality of care provided to children under five years of age at health facility and household levels; (b) strengthen the health system in order to sustain IMCI implementation; (c) empower communities to improve community and family practices to prevent child morbidity and mortality.

Expanded Program on immunization (EPI). The five-year EPI national strategic action plan is divided into 3 sections: (a) strengthen and implement routine activities, (b) organize supplemental immunization activities, and (c) strengthen integrated disease surveillance system and conduct active AFP (all suspected cases of polio) surveillance. Its goals for 2004 are to: (a) achieve and maintain immunization coverage of at least 90 percent for all antigens, (b) reduce measles morbidity by 90 percent and mortality by 95 percent compared with pre-immunization levels, (c) reduce the rate of neonatal tetanus (NNT) to less than 1 case per 1,000 live births with 100 percent reporting in all zones, (d) eradicate polio by 2000, and (e) introduce Hepatitis B vaccine with EPI routing by 2000.

Reproductive Health Program. This program includes: (a) safe motherhood (prenatal care, safe delivery, essential obstetric care, peri-natal and neonatal care, postnatal care and breastfeeding); (b) family planning information and services; (c) prevention and management of infertility and sexual dysfunction in both men and women; (d) prevention and management of abortion complications and provision of safe abortion services; (e) prevention and management of reproductive tract infections, especially STD's and HIV/AIDS; (f) promotion of healthy sexual maturation from pre-adolescence, responsible and safe sex throughout life, and gender equality; (g) elimination of harmful practices such as female genital mutilation (FGM), premature marriage and domestic and sexual violence against women; and (h) management of non-infectious conditions of the reproductive system such as cervical cancer, complications of FGM, etc.

The program seeks to develop a comprehensive program to reduce maternal mortality, improve the quality of antenatal care, and improve the use of family planning services. Attention will be focused on improving the quality of comprehensive reproductive care at all levels and on integrating reproductive services with child health services.

Nutrition. The long-term objectives of the nutrition program are to improve the nutritional status of the population especially women and children, and to ensure food security in all households. The Nutrition program is comprised of five sub-programs that deal with: (i) integrated PHC services, (ii) micronutrients which cover initiatives to reduce deficiencies in IDD, vitamin A, and iron, (iii) breastfeeding and complementary feeding; (iv) school health, and (v) food security and related strategies. The short-term goals for 2003 are to: (a) eliminate iodine deficiency disorders (IDD), (b) eliminate vitamin A deficiency, (c) reduce iron deficiency anemia by 33 percent, (d) achieve national food security, and (e) incorporate food and nutrition objectives within health, agriculture, poverty alleviation, education, industry and other sectoral priorities.

Environmental Health. The strategies and activities adopted under environmental health will emphasize the following areas: (a) prevention of diarrhea and intestinal parasite infestations through: excreta containment, water source protection and handling, maintenance and use of safe water, and food safety and hygiene; (b) prevention of ARI through interventions that reduce indoor air pollution, and include promotion of fuel-efficient stoves, substitution of biomass levels, promotion of improved kitchen/household ventilation; (c) collaboration in the prevention of malaria and other vector borne diseases through environment impact assessments, residual spraying, personal protection such as insecticide impregnated bed nets, and larvacides; (d) prevention of accidents in residences and public areas, (e) continuous hygiene education aimed at all community members, and (f) collaboration and coordination at the community, sub-zoba, zoba and national levels.

Information, Education, and Communication (IEC). The aims of IEC are to: (a) rationalize planning coordination and implementation of IEC for health promotion, (b) expand and strengthen partnerships for health promotion to increase the research of IEC efforts and their effectiveness, and (c) strengthen the health promotion infrastructure of MOH and its capacity to plan and deliver audience-based IEC activities at all levels.

Community Health Services (CHS). MOH is responsible for training community health workers (CHWs), providing refresher courses, technical assistance, continuous supportive supervision and monitoring, and providing CHWs with initial medical supplies and drugs to start the CHS programs. Communities are responsible for electing CHWs who will serve them. They are also responsible for remunerating them and providing them with a work place, furniture, equipment, and drugs after the initial medical supplies and drugs provided by MOH have been utilized. The community also decides whether drugs will be sold or given to patients for free, or at a subsidized rate. The CHS program seeks to: (a) enhance the links between conventional health services and community; (b) facilitate training of CHWs by training trainers and preparing training manuals; (c) establish mechanisms that encourage communities to take responsibility for their own health and be involved in planning, implementation and evaluation of health services; (d) improve community understanding of the health services system and how CHWs can improve the health of the community; (e) facilitate establishment and active involvement of health committees at every level; (f) enable health workers at all levels to support the implementation of the program; (g) promote sustainability of the program; (h) increase the number of births attended by trained birth attendants; (i) improve the technical support systems for provision of supplies, supervision, and referral, and (j) strengthen supportive supervision, monitoring and evaluation.

B. Communicable Diseases Control

The Division of Communicable Disease Control has the following units:

Malaria Control Unit. This unit is responsible for the implementation of MOH malaria control strategy which emphasizes case management, epidemic management and control, environmental control and selective vector control. An integrated health service approach is used in supervising the implementation of this strategy which is endorsed by WHO Roll Back Malaria Program. It involves early detection and prompt treatment of malaria cases, decreasing human-mosquito contact and protecting patients during medical procedures such as blood transfusions.

Tuberculosis Control Unit. This unit seeks to reduce morbidity, mortality, transmission and resistance to treatment throughout the country by training health personnel, increasing the number of properly equipped health facilities, enforcing uninterrupted drug treatment, and improving diagnostic capabilities. It is implementing the WHO treatment strategy of Directly Observed Treatment Short Course (DOTS).

Quarantine and Epidemics Control. This program aims to prevent epidemics and to monitor their outbreak, as well as the transmission of infectious diseases, to improve sanitation around the ports and to prevent the spread of disease vectors by developing appropriate legislation and quarantine strategies.

After the resolution of African Nations to strengthen Integrated Disease Surveillance, MOH is planning to implement the program in Eritrea. IDS is mainly concerned with regular collection of data and flow of information on selected priority diseases for surveillance purposes.

HIV/AIDS and STD Control. This program seeks to curb the spread of HIV/AIDS primarily through behavioral change. The main components of the strategy are behavioral change, STI control, community mobilization, voluntary counseling and testing and condom promotion.

Clinical Services

The Division of Clinical Services is responsible for the supervision of diagnostic, curative, and rehabilitative services which complement the preventive and promotive aspects of PHC. It oversees the provision of health care and supervises the treatment and care given in all the health facilities of MOH. It also collaborates with associations of health professionals to regulate professional conduct.

The division is also responsible for the development of policy and guidelines for medical practice, in accordance with MOH Quality Assurance Program. It has three units: (1) Medical Services Unit which is primarily responsible for supervision of diagnostic and curative services, (2) the Treatment and Care Unit which focuses on nursing services, and (3) the Licensing Unit which primarily deals with the licensing of private clinical practice.

Department of Pharmaceutical Services

The Department of Pharmaceutical Services is responsible for the implementation and monitoring of the National Drug Policy. Its basic functions include developing policies and guidelines, control of narcotic and psychotropic substances, drug information, and drug quality control. The department has two divisions:

Drug Control which is responsible for the enforcement of national and international regulations pertaining to drugs including narcotics, psychotropic and other controlled substances, inspection and licensing drug outlets and quality control of drugs.

Drug Management which aims to ensure effective drug management and rational drug use at all levels. It also aims to improve overall logistics management by designing a drug consumption reporting system especially for the primary levels of health service.

Division of Research and Human Resources Department

This division is responsible for the improvement of health services through development of human resources for health, research, and provision of accurate, timely and relevant information for informed decisions and interventions. It consists of five units, three of which involve Human Resource/training activities.

Training which is responsible for pre-service education of health professionals, particularly that of middle cadre health workers.

Continuing Education which is responsible for capacity building and upgrading of MOH staff.

Human Resources Planning which is charged with the development of a Strategic Human resource Development Plan for Health and for the monitoring and evaluation of HRD programs.

Research which seeks to institute regulatory mechanisms for health research, strengthen research capability of health workers and nurture a research culture. It also coordinates and conduct health related research. Some of the main achievements of this Unit are the following: (a) development and ratification of Health Research Policy and Guidelines, (b) identification of priority health research topics in Eritrea, (c) establishment of a central medical library and zonal satellite libraries, and (d) conducting and facilitating research on various topics include a collaborative project with the University of Leeds on the Practice of Strategic Planning in Health Sector Reform.

Some of its future activities include: conducting further training in health systems research methodology to build a critical mass of health workers capable of conducing research independently; organization of annual health research days, publication of the Health Policy Research Policy and National Health Research Priorities for Eritrea, and establishment of an Internet service in the Medical Library to facilitate literature searches.

Health Management Information Systems (HMIS) which aims to provide accurate, relevant and timely information to help make informed decisions and interventions. Some of its main achievements include: establishment of a network of data collection, processing and dissemination, computerization of data entry and processing up to the zonal level, publication of Annual Health Service Activity Reports since 1998, and development and installation of Local Area Network and Wide Area Network Programs to expedite data and information transfer, and training of health workers in data collection and use. Future plans include: development of a computerized Decision Support System for MOH and development of a Health Information website for the Worldwide Web.

National Laboratory Services

The national health laboratory structure of Eritrea is based on a three-tier system of peripheral, intermediate/regional, and central hospital laboratories, with the Central Health laboratory as the national reference. The Central Health Laboratory includes standardization of test methods, development of new technologies, implementation and monitoring of national quality control (include external proficiency testing) programs, in-service training of technical staff by conducting workshops and other forms of training. As a preliminary step towards quality accreditation, the laboratory participates in international external quality control programs.

Laboratory tests in hospitals tend to be limited to rudimentary, simple routine tests. For example, microbiology culture and sensitivity, histology and cytology, most immuno-serology and clinical chemistry laboratory tests are performed in the Central Health Laboratory only. While this has served the country's needs to date, it is insufficient to support the momentum of expanding national health services. Issues related to shortages in personnel, equipment and supplies; need for training and standardized internal quality control and preventive maintenance and repair, and lack of networking across different levels of health services facilities would need to be addressed (MOH 1999).

According to the Head of HRD, an in-depth study of laboratory services in Eritrea will be undertaken shortly.

GEOGRAPHIC DISTRIBUTION OF HEALTH FACILITIES IN ERITREA IN YEAR 2000

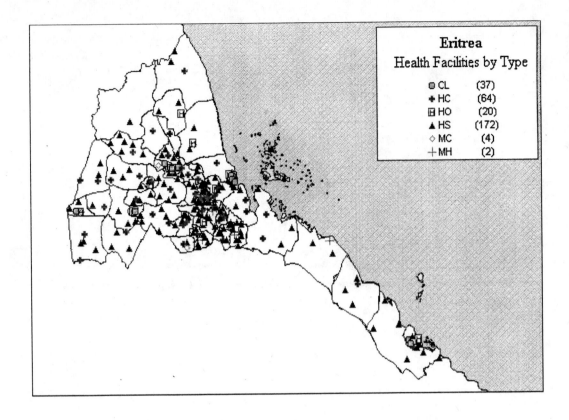

HEALTH CARE FINANCING[26]

Table E1 and Figure E1 show results from a study capturing some public sector and some private sector spending towards health care. Table E1 and Figure E1 provides break-down of the total health spending between the public and private sectors, and by donor contribution. Table E2 and Figures E2, E3, and E4 give a historical trend of MOH expenditures.

MOH Expenditures—Historical Trends

Estimates of low, medium, and high scenarios of aggregate public health sector costs and financing from all sources (in real 2001 Nakfa) for the next 5 years indicate a financing gap between the projected costs of the health sector, and available financing from government combined with donor recurrent budget support. According to Table E3, The low scenario projects a shortfall of Nafka 58.1 million of a total budgeted cost of Nafka 204.7 million by 2007 (in real 2001 terms), the medium scenario projects a shortfall of Nafka 27.4 million of a total budgeted cost of Nafka 230.9 million by 2007 (in real 2001 terms), and the high scenario projects a shortfall of Nafka 12.1 million of a total budgeted cost of Nafka 269.8 million by 2007 (in real 2001 terms, 000).[27]

---

26. This Annex is mainly based on Donaldson (2000). Further economic and financial analysis is being undertaken as part of Step 2 of the HSN process.

27. The low scenario assumes a low rate of real GDP growth (1 percent), the medium scenario assumes a moderate rate of GDP growth (3 percent), and the high scenario assumes a high rate of growth (7 percent). The other key variables influencing health sector costs were rates of population growth and changes in the number of hospital beds. On the financing side, the same GDP assumptions applied to government budgetary resources for health, and increasing per capita levels of donor financing were assumed. User fee revenue was generally assumed to grow with GDP and population growth, although the "high" scenario assumed an ambitious target of collecting fees equivalent to 1 percent of GDP by 2010.

TABLE E.1: ERITREA, HEALTH SPENDING ESTIMATES IN NOMINAL NAFKA AND PERCENT, 1999

Expenditure categories	Amount (Nakfa in millions)	Percent
Capital costs	24.0	14%
Government	9.0	5%
Donor	15.0	9%
Recurrent costs	133.3	78%
Government	103.2	60%
Donor	30.1	18%
Household Expenditure 1/	13.6	8%
TOTAL (Nafka, millions)	**170.8**	**100%**
Per capita (Nafka)	48.8	

Source: Donaldson, Dayl, Technical Report, *Economic and Financial Analysis,* September 2000.
1/   Household expenditure was estimated as follows: 3.5 million persons, 4.4 persons per household (DHS, 1997), mean health expenditure from all EHHSUES' households = N 17.1. It is worth noting that these estimates are actually below the reported government revenue from fees for 1999 of Nakfa 15,427,963, which implies that households paid more in 1999 for health than in 1997. Since these fees do not result in additional expenditures of the sector, it may not be appropriate to include them in NHA estimates.
Note: Figures are rounded off.

Donaldson (2002) proposes the following actions to address the above scenarios and bridge the financing gap:

Low Scenario: The size of the recurrent financing gap in this scenario is due to the addition of 400 beds, low provision of donor financial support, and low economic growth providing increases in government financing. Ways to narrow this gap include: reviewing the bed and other capacity needs of existing and future infrastructure, re-doubling efforts to identify donor recurrent financing, and seeking ways to increase user fee revenue and require that it be budgeted as part of the existing level of government financial support to the sector.

FIGURE E.1: ERITREA, SOURCE OF HEALTH CARE FINANCING, 1999 (PERCENT)

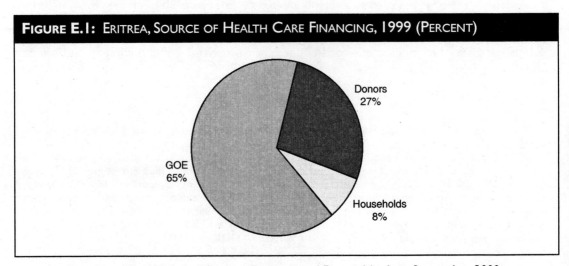

Source: Donaldson, Dayl, Technical Report, *Economic and Financial Analysis,* September 2000.

TABLE E.2: ERITREA, PUBLIC SECTOR REVIEW OF HEALTH, 1995–1999 (IN NOMINAL AND REAL NAFKA)

Expenditure categories	1995 Nafka	%	1996 Nafka	%	1997 Nafka	%	1998 Nafka	%	1999 Nafka	%
Capital costs										
Govt.					5,428,578		5,578,664		8,966,737	
Donor	6,365,283	100	19,111,423	100	10,348,789	65.6	20,714,850	78.8	15,010,258	62.6
Total—Nominal	6,365,283		19,111,423		15,777,368		26,293,515		23,976,995	
Total—Real '92 Nafka	4,951,216		14,307,099		11,606,980		16,590,015		13,968,538	
% Annual Change			189		−18.9		42.9		−15.8	
Recurrent costs										
Govt.	80,347,849		58,242,030		82,102,321		96,036,663		103,170,555	
Salary	61,304,213	66.7	32,264,164	51.7	53,742,339	51.0	58,930,907	50.2	63,487,006	47.6
Drugs	9,074,440	9.9	12,601,639	20.2	1,313,2180	12.5	18,030,014	15.4	1,659,6164	12.5
Other	9,971,197	10.9	13,376,227	21.4	15,227,803	14.5	19,075,742	16.2	23,087,384	17.3
Donor	11,501,778		4,183,542		23,211,672		21,356,439		30,072,373	
Salary										
Drugs	10,181,056	11.1	2,142,680	3.4	510,2629	4.8	11,377,111	9.7	18,386,680	13.8
Other										
Non-specified	1,320,722	1.4	2,040,862	3.3	18,109,043	17.2	9,979,328	8.5	11,685,693	8.8
Total nominal	91,849,627	100	62,425,572	100	10,531,3993	100	117,393,102	100	133,242,927	100
Total—Real '92 Nafka	71,444,950		46,732,723		77,476,637		7,406,9721		77,624,776	
% Annual Change			−34.6		65.8		−4.4		4.8	
Revenue										
Registration Fees							10,604,399	78.8	12,739,858	82.6
Drug Fees							2,745,486	20.4	2,569,318	16.7
Other							110,088	0.8	118,788	0.8
Total—Nominal	3,704,223		8,325,239		12,164,203		13459,973	100	15,427,963	100
% of Recurrent	4%		13.3		11.6		11.5		11.6	
Total—Real '92 Nafka	288,1318		6,232,399		8,948,873		8,492,632		8,988,036	
% Annual Change			1,16.3		43.6		−5.1		5.8	
CPI (1992 = 100)	12,8.56		13,3.58		13,5.93		15,8.93		171.65	

Source: Finance Office, MOH, cited in Donaldson, Dayl. Technical Report, Economic and Financial Analysis, September 2000.
[2]*Note: Salary figures include back-payments to fighters.*

Medium Scenario: The results of this scenario in terms of higher levels of costs (and presumably more health services) and financing, provide greater flexibility in developing and adopting a revised user fee policy. The objectives of the policy should be to match the growth of fee revenue to the growth of the economy and the growth of utilization (proxied by the growth of the population).

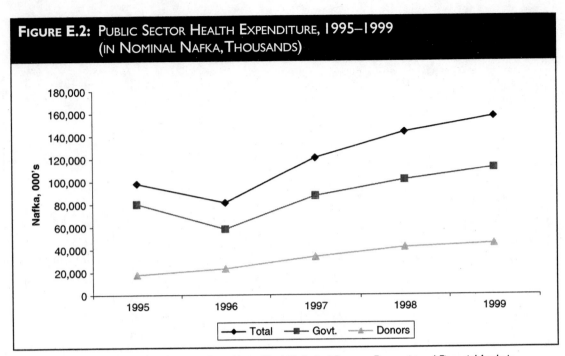

FIGURE E.2: PUBLIC SECTOR HEALTH EXPENDITURE, 1995–1999 (IN NOMINAL NAFKA, THOUSANDS)

Source: Finance Office, MOH, cited in Donaldson, Dayl. Technical Report, *Economic and Financial Analysis,* September 2000.

High Scenario: The results of the high scenario should be regarded as upper limits for the expansion of the costs and financing for the sector. Given historical rates of economic growth in sub-Saharan Africa it is unclear that Eritrea will achieve an average annual real rate of GDP growth of 7 percent. It is also difficult to predict the trend in donor financing for the sector and the real per capita level of donor financing may not remain constant considering population

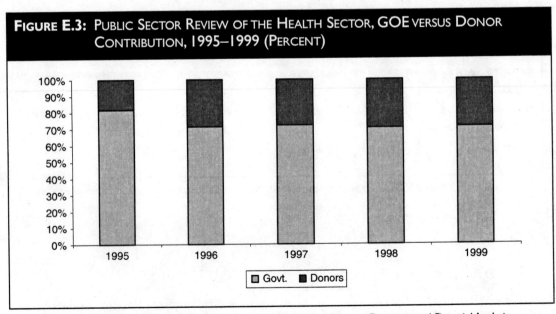

FIGURE E.3: PUBLIC SECTOR REVIEW OF THE HEALTH SECTOR, GOE VERSUS DONOR CONTRIBUTION, 1995–1999 (PERCENT)

Source: Finance Office, MOH, cited in Donaldson, Dayl. Technical Report, *Economic and Financial Analysis,* September 2000.

TABLE E.3: MOH FINANCING PROJECTION RESULTS, 2001–2007, REAL 2001 NAKFA ('000)

	Year						
	2001	**2002**	**2003**	**2004**	**2005**	**2006**	**2007**
Projections							
Low							
Recurrent	208,198	187,759	193,824	200,008	201,539	203,079	204,682
Government + donor revenue	208,198	136,241	138,225	140,246	142,303	144,398	146,531
Revenue-cost	0	–51,519	–55,599	–59,762	–59,236	–58,699	–58,151
User fees	15,607	16,169	16,751	17,354	17,979	18,626	19,297
Medium							
Recurrent	208,198	199,937	208,845	217,474	221,763	226,223	230,862
Government + donor revenue	208,198	177,049	182,050	187,192	192,480	197,919	203,512
Revenue-cost	0	–22,887	–26,435	–30,282	–29,282	–28,304	–27,350
User fees	15,607	16,403	17,240	18,119	19,043	20,014	21,035
High							
Recurrent	208,198	213,216	225,806	239,692	248,986	258,989	269,760
Government + donor revenue	208,198	201,841	211,627	221,895	232,953	244,569	257,688
Revenue-cost	0	–11,735	–14,179	–17,706	–16,033	–14,420	–12,072
User fees	15,607	20,055	25,771	33,115	42,553	54,681	70,265

FIGURE E.4: ERITREA, PUBLIC SECTOR REVIEW OF RECURRENT EXPENDITURE FOR HEALTH, 1995–1999 (PERCENT)

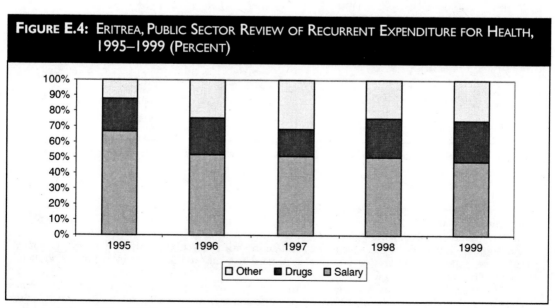

Source: Finance Office, MOH, cited in Donaldson, Dayl. Technical Report, *Economic and Financial Analysis,* September 2000.

growth. Moreover while it is feasible that the population, on average, could pay 1 percent of GDP for health services, it is unlikely that the public sector will be able to mobilize this level of fee collection without altering access and quality of service.

Costs of Health Services

Unit Cost Analysis

Unit costs of health services are not readily available. This section uses results from a study by Yoder (1995),[28] which was conducted over six years ago in 1996.[29] Table E4 provides the estimated average unit costs of selected services provided by the sample facilities in 1994. The unit cost estimates for visits to government health centers and stations were higher for inpatient care, but lower for outpatient visits. Estimates suggest that an inpatient day unit cost would be Nafka 1,261 to 4,115 at health centers and health stations respectively, compared to Nafka 82 at provincial hospitals, and an outpatient visit unit cost would range between Nafka 15 to 31 at health centers and health stations respectively, compared to Nafka 36 at provincial hospitals in 1994[30]. There was considerable variability in the actual point estimates for individual facilities, which suggests that using unit cost figures to set user fees, or project recurrent costs of facilities, may require utilizing a range of estimates, rather than one average figure. Moreover, the high average unit costs at health centers and health stations as compared to hospitals suggests that utilization is low relative to the fixed costs of these facilities. Further, more recent cost studies will be required.

TABLE E.4: UNIT COST ESTIMATES IN NAFKA FOR HEALTH FACILITIES BY TYPE OF SERVICE, 1994[31]

Type of health services	Provincial hospitals (3)	Health centers (4)	Health stations (8)	Average all facilities (15)
IP Bed day	82	1,261	4,115	1,164
Delivery	2,536	6,861	5,875	4,992
OP visit	36	31	15	23
Immunization	63	225	110	153
FP visit	2,663	1,470	4,725	3,758
Growth monitoring	141	146	308	226
Child visit	188	244	89	145
Antenatal visit	237	612	602	553
Lab exam	422	508	NA	457

Source: Yoder, R. *Eritrean Health and Population Project, Health Facilities Cost Estimates Study*, BASICS Project. 1995.

---

28. Yoder (1995) calculated the cost of delivering out-patient (OPD) health services at health stations, health center, and at the OPDs of provincial hospitals. The sample size was 15 health facilities selected through a cluster sampling methodology used in four areas of Eritrea.

29. Another study estimates that the unit cost of an in-patient day at government (tertiary?) hospitals were Birr 54, and outpatient visits at government tertiary hospitals were Birr 18. Source of this study is unknown. This study was cited in World Bank (1997).

30. No references were found which estimate the capitated cost of a primary health care package of services.

31. Care must be taken in the use of these unit cost estimates, as they reflect the "technology" and services being provided in 1994 which would affect total costs, and the size and composition of the market which would affect utilization.

Cost-effectiveness of Public Sector Health Interventions

A burden of disease (BOD), and a cost-effectiveness (CE) study was carried out in 1994 (Sebhatu 1994). This study calculated the burden of disease from 10 disease groups (which were estimated to account for 59 percent of total deaths and 73 percent of the discounted years of life lost in Eritrea), and then the cost-effectiveness of community, preventive and curative interventions to reduce the burden of disease from these illnesses. The cost-effectiveness ratios for these interventions appear in Table E5.[32] The results recommend a preventive or community treatment intervention for 9 out of the 10 diseases.

The BOD/CE study also relates the share of government expenditure for a particular disease to the share of BOD contributed by the specific illness. The results of this analysis are presented in Table E6. The study analysis suggests that financial resources for the health sector should be reallocated to better match the share of BOD, and towards interventions which are more cost-effective. For example, diarrheal diseases, and immunizable diseases contribute significantly to the BOD, but receives a lower proportionate share of health expenditure.[33]

The BOD/CE study also proposes a policy package of cost sharing, privatization, and decentralization. While these policies do not follow from the findings of the BOD/CE study, these may be considered on their own merits, and will be taken up in other sections of this report.

TABLE E.5: COST-EFFECTIVENESS OF DISEASE INTERVENTIONS (BIRR/DISCOUNTED LIFE YEAR SAVED)

	Community	Preventive	Curative
Malaria	753	1,438	67 *
ARI	19 *	113	31
Perinatal/Maternal	11 *	105	8 *
Nutritional deficiency	11 *	203	415
Diarrea	11 *	84	124
Cardiovascular	NA	1,501 *	6,901
AIDS/STDs	2,605	165 *	7,436
Immunizable disease	11	5 *	29
Tuberculosis	11 *	18 *	153
Injury/Trauma	NA	NA	50
All other disease	655	203 *	2,644

Source: Sebhatu, M. et.al. "Eritrea, Summary Report" In: *Proceedings of the East Africa Burden of Disease, Cost-Effectiveness of Health Care Interventions and Health Policy.* Regional Workshop, August 17–19, 1994.

Note: * Indicates a recommended intervention.

32. There are several limitations to this study, which the authors acknowledge. These include failure to include: the burden of disease from the disability arising from any of the illness, disabling chronic illnesses such as diabetes and hepatitis, the externality and synergistic benefits from community or preventive interventions, and the costs of transport for curative services. The authors also recognize that the poor quality of data limit the validity of the results. In addition, the study calculates point estimates of cost effectiveness without providing information as to the scale for each intervention (i.e., is it the cost-effectiveness ratio related to a national program?).

33. This example points to another of the limitations of the study, namely that investments in improving water supply and sanitation are not included in health expenditure, but would certainly contribute to reducing the burden of disease from diarrhea.

TABLE E.6: SHARE OF BURDEN OF DISEASES VERSUS SHARE OF BUDGETARY SPENDING, 1994

	% Share of BOD		% Share of spending
Malaria	5.56	<	6.97
ARI	14.70	>	12.86
Perinatal/Maternal	17.87	>	15.27
Nutritional Deficiency	2.24	>	1.88
Diarrhea	17.40	>	3.03
Cardiovascular	1.62	>	0.64
AIDS/STDs	1.93	<	2.06
Immunizable Disease	4.40	>	0.27
Tuberculosis	7.13	>	4.23
Injury/Trauma	0.59	<	5.94
All Other Causes	26.57	<	46.85

Source: Sebhatu, M. et.al. "Eritrea, Summary Report". In: Proceedings of the East Africa Burden of Disease, Cost-Effectiveness of Health Care Interventions and Health Policy. Regional Workshop, August 17–19, 1994.

TABLE E.7: PERCENT OF HOUSEHOLDS REPORTING AN ILLNESS WHO MADE VARIOUS LEVELS OF PAYMENT BY TYPE OF EXPENDITURE, 1997

Expenditure amount (Nakfa)	Percent of people paying					
	Registration	Drugs	X-ray	Room	Transport	Other
0	35%	53%	95%	96%	86%	95%
1–50	34%	43%	6%	3%	13%	4%
51–100	22%	3%	0.2%	0.4%	1%	0.4%
101+	9%	2%	NA	0.4%	0.2%	0.8%
Total	100	100	100	100	100	100

Source: Eritrea Household Health Status, Utilization and Expenditures Survey (EHHSUES), 1997.
NA = Not Available / Not Applicable.

Health Care Expenditures and Payment Methods

Fee for service is the most common payment method used for health care. However, health care fees are heavily subsidized by the Government at MOH health facilities. Health insurance is almost non-existent.

Table E7 shows that most patients paid for health care. Thirty-five percent of health facility users paid no registration fees while 9 percent of users paid over Nafka 100. However, the report did not indicate the total amount paid by households for all treatments/inputs used for the illness reported. The results suggest however that the majority of the population pay little for treatment aside from a registration fee and drugs[34].

---

34. The report does not give a distribution of households' expenditures for drugs.

TABLE E.8: HOUSEHOLD CONSUMPTION AND HEALTH EXPENDITURES AMONG TOTAL SAMPLE HOUSEHOLDS AND AMONG HOUSEHOLDS UTILIZING HEALTH FACILITIES, 1997

	Households with health facility in town or village	Households with no health facility in town or village	Total sample
All HHs			
Estimated Household Monthly Consumption (Nakfa)	562.6	377.5	427.4
Estimated Monthly Health Expenditure (Nakfa)	11.2	15.1	17.1
% of Consumption	2%	4%	4%
HHs Using Health Facility			
Estimated Household Monthly Consumption (Nakfa)	624.2	399.3	456.7
Estimated Household Monthly Health Expenditure (Nakfa)	37.4	39.9	41.1
% of Consumption	6%	10%	9%

Source: *Eritrea Household Health Status, Utilization and Expenditures Survey* (EHHSUES), 1997.

The EHHSUES study showed that on average, households spend about 4 percent of their average monthly consumption (Nakfa 11 per household per month) on health services. Of only those households reporting illness, expenditure for health was about 6 percent of total household consumption (Nakfa 28 per household per month), and this probably did not include travel and pharmaceutical costs. A study by Weaver (1997) reanalyzed some of the EHHSUES data to estimate the proportion of household income that was spent for health. Table E8 shows that households with health facility in town or village are relatively better off compared to households with no health facility in town or village. On a per capita basis, the estimated monthly health expenditure was more or less the same between these two groups, Nafka 37 for those with health facility, and Nafka 40 for those with health facility. However, households without health facility who were also better-off spent on average about 6 percent of household consumption compared to the less fortunate who spent 10 percent of household consumption on health care on a monthly basis. Compare to literature from developing countries which show that poor household could be spending from 3 to 5 percent of their household consumption on health, poor Eritrean households may be spending a lot on health care. The MOH is embarking on new pricing and cost recovery strategies, a closer look will be required of its effects on consumers, and particularly the poor and the vulnerable groups[35].

New Proposed Health Care Pricing Policy at MOH

In February 1996, the MOH introduced user fees (registration fees, and daily hotel fees) at all public health facilities. The fees were introduced in order to: 1) provide substantial subsidies for primary care, 2) charge patients the full costs of care at tertiary facilities, and 3) encourage patients to use the referral system appropriately. Table E9 gives the referred and the by-pass prices charged at the MOH health facilities, and the percent of unit costs recovered from

---

35. Donaldson (2000) recommends that, based on current findings from Eritrea, the scope for increasing health fees be restricted to the higher income households in Eritrea.

TABLE E.9: PERCENT OF UNIT COSTS RECOVERED THROUGH USER FEE POLICY BY MOH HEALTH FACILITIES, 1996

Health facility level	Referred price in nafka	Bypass price in nafka	Percent of unit cost recovered
Hospital-OP/Visit	7	16	18 to 36
Hospital-IP Day	9.5	19	54 to 82
Health Center-OP/Visit	5	8	31
Health Station-OP/Visit	3	NA	15

Source: SOE/MOH. *Health Care Financing Policy*, Asmara : MOH, October 1999.
NA = Not Applicable/Not Available.

revenue. In 1996, on average, 11 percent of MOH health recurrent costs were recovered through user fees.

In 1998, MOH developed a new Health Care Financing Policy. The policy has not been implemented to date because of the difficult situation during the war with Ethiopia. The policy is designed to revise the user charges for different categories of patients, and has dealt with exemption scheme issues, and cost assessments of different health services as a basis for fee calculations. The document also reviews the different areas of health insurance and concludes that an insurance scheme would be difficult to implement in Eritrea, partly due to the low demand from and low awareness of the population to health care costs. Table E10 provides the proposed schedule for user fees at the different levels of the health system.

The objectives of this new financing policy are to achieve the following targets:

- Increase revenue by 200 percent over current levels;
- Improve the efficiency, equity, and quality of health care;
- Create incentives for patients to use preventive and PHC services as first entry points into the health care system;
- Encourage the community to become more responsible and self-reliant for their own health care.
- To ensure efficient collection of user fees, and to ensure the proper use of revenue from user fees, MOH has outlined the following proposed policies:
- MOH Health centers and stations will retain 30 percent of revenue collected;
- MOH Hospitals will retain 20 percent of revenue collected;
- The Zonal Health Office will retain 10 percent of the revenue collected; and
- The remaining revenue will be transferred to the Central Treasury, Ministry of Finance.
- Retained fees may be used solely for the purchase of supplies and facility maintenance, but not for the purchase of drugs or for providing financial incentives to employees.

The health financing policy document estimated that the application of the new fee schedule at the MOH health facilities, would increase the annual earnings from Nakfa 17 million to approximately Nafka 52 million, or by 206 percent.[36]

---

36. This estimated amount is simply the current level of about 17 million, plus an additional 200 percent.

TABLE E.10: SCHEDULE OF USER FEES AT DIFFERENT HEALTH FACILITY LEVELS

Type of patient	Hospital	Health center	Health station 3/
Ordinary citizens 1/	50% labor cost	65% labor cost	70% labor cost
	100% consumables	100% of non-hotel	100% of non-hotel
	30% equipment cost	operating costs	operating costs
	100% hotel cost	Nafka 3.00/day	105% drug cost
	110% drug cost	110% drug cost	
		lab fees according	
		to price list	
Service on credit	75% labor cost		
	100% consumables		
	30% equipment		
	100% hotel cost		
	110% drug cost		
Insured citizens	100% of all costs		
Foreign citizens	100% labor cost		
	100% consumables		
	100% equipment		
	100% hotel cost		
	125% drug cost		
	100% ancillary services cost		
Expatriates 2/	200% labor		
	200% consumables		
	200% equipment		
	200% hotel cost		
	(+50% special accommodation)		
	140% drug cost		
	250% ancillary services cost		

Source: SOE/MOH. *Health Care Financing Policy,* Asmara : MOH, October 1999.

1/ At MOH hospitals, children are charged 50 percent of the registration, consultation, and hotel charges only.

2/ Payment is expected in US dollars.

3/ No exemptions will be provided for acute, curative health services at health stations as the services under the proposed pricing guidelines are believed to be highly subsidized.

Note: The policy specifies certain illnesses or services which will be exempt from fees. These are: antenatal services, well baby services, immunizations, leprosy, mental illness, STDs, HIV/AIDs, emergency cases for first 24 hours, injuries from explosives. In addition, those who can obtain a certificate of indigenous from the local MOLG office will receive free care. The costs of their care however will have to be paid by the local government which issued the certificate.

INTERNATIONAL COMPARISON TABLES

TABLE F.1: SUB-SAHARAN AFRICA, GLOBAL DEMOGRAPHIC INDICATORS, 1999

Country name	Population—1999	Growth (%) 1999	TFR—1999
Angola	12,356,900	2.88	6.68
Benin	6,114,050	2.75	5.60
Botswana	1,588,120	1.68	4.14
Burkina Faso	10,995,700	2.44	6.56
Burundi	6,677,950	1.96	6.08
Cameroon	14,690,500	2.67	4.86
Cape Verde	427,790	2.96	3.75
Central African Republic	3,539,810	1.70	4.74
Chad	7,485,610	2.75	6.32
Comoros	544,280	2.50	4.38
Congo, Dem. Rep.	49,775,500	3.18	6.24
Congo, Rep.	2,858,760	2.70	5.94
Cote d'Ivoire	15,545,500	2.57	4.94
Equatorial Guinea	442,680	2.58	5.33
Eritrea	3,991,000	2.85	5.56
Ethiopia	62,782,000	2.44	6.26
Gabon	1,208,410	2.35	5.08
Gambia, The	1,251,000	2.84	5.46
Ghana	18,784,500	2.27	4.26
Guinea	7,250,520	2.29	5.33
Guinea-Bissau	1,184,670	1.99	5.54
Kenya	29,410,000	2.13	4.51
Lesotho	2,105,000	2.27	4.51
Madagascar	15,050,500	3.09	5.56
Malawi	10,787,800	2.39	6.31
Mali	10,583,700	2.39	6.36
Mauritania	2,598,330	2.70	5.26
Mauritius	1,174,400	1.26	2.02
Mozambique	17,299,000	1.95	5.18
Namibia	1,701,330	2.33	4.73
Niger	10,495,600	3.39	7.28
Nigeria	123,897,000	2.52	5.21
Rwanda	8,310,000	2.50	5.98
Sao Tome and Principe	145,260	2.27	4.53
Senegal	9,285,310	2.69	5.44
Seychelles	80,030	1.49	2.10
Sierra Leone	4,949,340	1.93	5.87
Somalia	9,388,250	3.38	7.13

TABLE F.1: SUB-SAHARAN AFRICA, GLOBAL DEMOGRAPHIC INDICATORS, 1999 (CONTINUED)

Country name	Population—1999	Growth (%) 1999	TFR—1999
South Africa	42,106,200	1.69	2.92
Sudan	28,993,300	2.25	4.52
Swaziland	1,019,470	2.89	4.50
Tanzania	32,922,600	2.44	5.43
Togo	4,566,940	2.42	5.08
Uganda	21,479,300	2.75	6.36
Zambia	9881,210	2.21	5.38
Zimbabwe	11,903,700	1.82	3.61
Average	13,391,935	2.43	5.21

Source: World Bank, *World Development Indicators 2001*, Washington, D.C.

TABLE F.2: SUB-SAHARAN AFRICA: HEALTH INDICATORS (1990–1999)

Country	Infant mortality rate (1999)	Under-5 mortality rate (1999)	Maternal mortality rate (1990–7)	Life exp. at birth (1999)
Angola	127	208	1,500	47
Benin	87	145	500	53
Botswana	58	95	250	39
Burkina Faso	105	210	930	45
Burundi	105	176	1,300	42
Cameroon	77	154	550	51
Central African Republic	96	151	700	44
Chad	101	189	840	49
Congo, Dem. Rep.	85	161	870	46
Congo, Rep.	89	144	890	48
Cote d'Ivoire	111	180	810	46
Djibouti	109	177	570	47
Equatorial Guinea	104	170		51
Eritrea	**60**	**105**	**1,000**	**50**
Ethiopia	104	180	1,400	42
Gabon	84	133	500	53
Gambia, The	75	110	1,050	53
Ghana	57	109	740	58
Guinea	96	167	880	46
Guinea-Bissau	127	214	910	44
Kenya	76	118	650	48
Lesotho	92	141	610	45
Madagascar	90	149	500	54
Malawi	132	227	620	39
Mali	120	223	580	43
Mauritania	88	142	800	54
Mauritius	19	23	110	71
Mozambique	131	203	1,100	43
Namibia	63	108	220	50
Niger	116	252	590	46
Nigeria	83	151	1,000	47
Rwanda	123	203	1,300	40
Sao Tome and Principe	47	66		65
Senegal	67	124	510	52
Seychelles	9	15		72

TABLE F.2: SUB-SAHARAN AFRICA: HEALTH INDICATORS (1990–1999) (CONTINUED)

Country	Infant mortality rate (1999)	Under-5 mortality rate (1999)	Maternal mortality rate (1990–7)	Life exp. at birth (1999)
Sierra Leone	168	283		37
South Africa	62	76	230	48
Sudan	67	109	370	56
Swaziland	64	113		46
Tanzania	95	152	530	45
Togo	77	143	640	49
Uganda	88	162	550	42
Zambia	114	187	650	38
Zimbabwe	70	118	280	40
Africa Region Average=	89.35	151.31	715.25	48.78

Source: World Bank, *World Development Indicators 2001*, Washington, D.C.

TABLE F.3: Sub-Saharan Africa, Physicians and Beds per 1,000 Population (1990–1999)

Country	Physicians per 1,000 population (1999)	Beds per 1,000 population (1998)
Angola	0.04	1.29
Benin	0.03	0.23
Botswana	0.19	1.58
Burkina Faso	—	1.42
Burundi	0.06	0.66
Cameroon	0.06	2.55
Central African Republic	0.03	0.87
Chad	0.02	0.72
Comoros	0.09	2.76
Congo, Dem. Rep.	0.05	1.43
Congo, Rep.	0.21	3.35
Cote d'Ivoire	0.07	0.80
Djibouti	0.13	2.54
Equatorial Guinea	0.22	
Eritrea	**0.02**	**0.75**
Ethiopia	0.03	0.24
Gabon	0.23	3.19
Gambia, The	0.02	0.61
Ghana	—	1.46
Guinea	0.11	0.55
Guinea-Bissau	0.18	1.48
Kenya	0.04	1.65
Lesotho	0.04	
Madagascar	1.14	0.94
Malawi	0.03	1.34
Mali	0.06	0.24
Mauritania	0.06	0.67
Mauritius	0.86	3.07
Mozambique	—	0.87
Namibia	0.23	
Niger	0.03	0.12
Nigeria	0.19	1.67
Rwanda	0.04	1.65
Sao Tome and Principe	0.42	4.74

TABLE F.3: SUB-SAHARAN AFRICA, PHYSICIANS AND BEDS PER 1,000 POPULATION (1990–1999) (CONTINUED)

Country	Physicians per 1,000 population (1999)	Beds per 1,000 population (1998)
Senegal	0.04	0.40
Seychelles	1.03	
South Africa	0.62	
Sudan	0.10	1.09
Swaziland	0.08	
Tanzania	0.04	0.89
Togo	0.06	1.51
Zimbabwe	0.12	0.51
Africa Region Average=	0.17	1.37

Source: World Bank, *World Development Indicators 2001,* Washington, D.C.

TABLE F.4: SUB-SAHARAN AFRICA, HEALTH EXPENDITURE PATTERN, 1990–1998

Country	Per capita GDP, US$ (1998)	Per capita public sector health exp, US$ (1998)	Public sector health exp. % of GDP (1998)
Angola	1,272	50	3.90
Benin	388	6	1.60
Botswana	3,123	78	2.50
Burkina Faso	240	3	1.20
Burundi	134	0.80	0.60
Cameroon	608	6	1.00
Central African Republic	301	6	2.00
Chad	231	5	2.30
Comoros	374	12	3.10
Congo, Dem. Rep.			—
Congo, Rep.	701	14	2.00
Cote d'Ivoire	742	9	1.20
Equatorial Guinea	1,184	36	3.00
Eritrea	**173**	**5**	**2.90**
Ethiopia	107	2	1.70
Gabon	3,913	82	2.10
Gambia, The	343	7	1.90
Ghana	407	7	1.80
Guinea	506	11	2.20
Guinea-Bissau	222	2	1.10
Kenya	398	10	2.40
Lesotho	484	16	3.40
Madagascar	256	3	1.10
Malawi	165	5	2.80
Mali	251	5	2.10
Mauritania	396	6	1.40
Mauritius	3,512	63	1.80
Mozambique	230	6	2.80
Namibia	1,831	75	4.10
Niger	205	2	1.20
Nigeria	267	2	0.80
Rwanda	250	5	2.00
Sao Tome and Principe	345	21	6.10
Senegal	516	13	2.60
Seychelles	6,789	367	5.40

TABLE F.4: SUB-SAHARAN AFRICA, HEALTH EXPENDITURE PATTERN, 1990–1998 (CONTINUED)

Country	Per capita GDP, US$ (1998)	Per capita public sector health exp, US$ (1998)	Public sector health exp. % of GDP (1998)
Sierra Leone	138	1	0.90
South Africa	3,236	107	3.30
Sudan	370	3	0.70
Swaziland	1,232	33	2.70
Tanzania	267	3	1.30
Togo	317	4	1.30
Uganda	324	6	1.90
Zambia	335	12	3.60
Zimbabwe	757	22	2.90
Africa Region Average=	880.08	26.34	2.20

Source: World Bank, *World Development Indicators 2001*, Washington, D.C.

MILLENNIUM DEVELOPMENT GOALS PROGRESS STATUS

MDG	Global Target(s)	Current Status	GOE Target	On/Off Track to Achieving Global and/or GOE Target
1: Eradicate extreme poverty and hunger	To halve, between 1990 and 2015, the proportion of people (i) with income of less than one dollar; and (ii) the proportion of people who suffer from hunger.	(i) 60–70% of the population is classified as living in poverty; one estimate is 53%. (ii) unemployment rate in the non-farm sectors is between 15–20%. (iii) 44% of children under the age of 5 years are underweight primarily due to insufficient food intake.	20–22%	(i) Off track
2: Achieve universal primary education	Ensure that, by 2015, children everywhere, boys and girls alike, will be able to complete a full course of primary schooling.	(i) NER for grades 1–5 is 33%. (ii) In 1999, net enrollment rate for children in primary school was 31 for girls and 36 for boys. (iii) (70%) of pupils who start primary school do not reach grade 5. (iv) 70% overall literacy rate for youth (15–24 years) illiteracy rate is 41% for female and 21% for males.	(i) 100% (ii) illiteracy rate reduced to 10%	(i) Off track (ii) On track
3: Promote gender equality and empower women	Eliminate gender disparity in primary and secondary education, preferably by 2005, and to all levels of education no later than 2015.	(i) gender parity at primary school level—ratio of girls to boys in primary school. is around 90%. (ii) gender disparity at secondary school level—17% rate for girls and 21% boys. (iii) Out of school youth—girls (72% for primary school and 66% for secondary. The comparable figures for boys are 69 and 59%).	100% by 2015	(i) Off track (ii) Off track

Goal	Target	Indicators	Status
		(iv) ratio of literate females to males aged 15–24 : 75%	
		(v) ratio of women to men in wage employment (non-agricultural sector) 47%.	
		(vi) 14.7% of seats in parliament occupied by women.	
4: Reduce child mortality	Reduce by two thirds, between 1990 and 2015, the under-five mortality rate	(i) IMR is 48 per 1000 live births.	(i) 27/1000 by year 2015 — (i) Off track
		(ii) 84% of children < 1year received measles vaccine.	(ii) 100% by 2015 — (ii) On track
5: Improve Maternal Health	Maternal Mortality Ratio (MMR)—reduce by 3/4 between 1990–2015	(i) MMR > 1000 per 100,000 live births	(i) 250,000 by 2015 — (i) Off track
		(ii) 28% of births attended by skilled personnel	
6: Combat HIV/AIDS, malaria and other diseases	By 2015 to have halted and begun to reverse, the spread of HIV/AIDS, (& other diseases e.g. malaria, TB)	(i) HIV adult sero-prevalence between 15 and 2.8%.	
		(ii) contraceptive rate: 8% of married women	
		(iii) TB: 50% diagnosed cases are smear-positive. Cure rate >60%.	Seems on track for HIV/AIDS
7: Ensure environmental sustainability	Halve, by 2015, the proportion of people without sustainable access to safe drinking water. By 2020, to have achieved a significant improvement in the lives of at least 100 million slum dwellers.	(i) Access to safe water: 8.1% of rural pop. & 59.6% in urban areas.	(i) By 2005 increase to 30% rural population with access to sanitation. — Seems off track
		(ii) Access to sanitation: 1% of rural population & 66% of urban population.	

ERITREA HEALTH SECTOR PERFORMANCE

Outline of Study Report

1. Introduction
    1.1   The health care system in Eritrea
    1.2   Performance of the health system: effectiveness and efficiency

2. Policy and Strategy Framework
    2.1   Health Sector Reform and Strategy
    2.2   Eritrea Health Sector Vision and Guiding Principles

3. The Pharmaceuticals Sector
    3.1   The National Drug Policy
    3.2   The Eritrean Drug Law
    3.3   The Eritrean National List of Drugs
    3.4   The Eritrean Standard Treatment Guidelines
    3.5   Organization of the Drug Administration, MOH
    3.6   Human resources
    3.7   Drug procurement
    3.8   Drug storage, distribution, and use of drugs
    3.9   The parastatal drug sector and PHARMECOR
    3.10 Erithro pharmaceutical factory, Keren
    3.11 The private pharmaceutical sector
    3.12 The National Drug Bill
    3.2   Drug accessibility, availability, and affordability
    3.3   Major problems and issues
    3.3   Future options

4. Health Care Financing
    4.1   The Health Financing Policy of 1996/98
    4.2   Levels and composition of financing
         4.2.1 Share of health sector expenditures in total national budget
         4.2.2 Public expenditure on health (evolution/trends, by category, by type, technical and economic efficiency)
         4.2.3 Resource allocations in the health sector (by region, by facility, by programs, efficiency and cost-effectiveness)
    4.3   Household health spending and services utilization patterns
         4.3.1 Household health spending and utilization by income quintiles and by health care provider (private/public/traditional)
         4.3.2 Household health spending and utilization by income quintiles and by health facility type
         4.3.3 Household health spending by health facility type and by region
         4.3.4 Household health spending by gender and age of household member
         4.3.5 Trends in household health spending and service utilization
         4.3.6 Determinants of household health spending and health service utilization
    4.4   Sources of financing
         4.4.1 Public revenues
         4.4.2 User fees (impact on growth of private sector, utilization of services, health facilities)
         4.4.3 Health insurance
         4.4.4 Other private sources
    4.5   Cost recovery

BIBLIOGRAPHY

College of Health Science. 2001. *Revised Curriculum of Bachelor of Pharmacy Program*, University of Asmara.

Department of Pharmaceutical Services, Ministry of Health of Eritrea. 2001. *Annual Report*. Asmara.

_____. 2000. *Annual Report 2000*. Asmara.

_____. 2001. Action Plan 2001. Asmara.

_____. 2002a. Essential Drugs & Medical Supplies, Logistics Management for Health Centers and Stations, 2nd ed.

_____. 2002b. Semi Annual Report. Asmara.

Donaldson, Daryl. 2000. *Technical Report: Economic and Financial Analysis*. Asmara: Ministry of Health.

_____. 2002. *Eritrea, Health Sector Investment and Financing Analyses*. Asmara: Ministry of Health.

Ewan Technology. 2001. *Integrated Information Systems Report for the Eritrea IECD Project*.

Government of Eritrea. 2001. Constitution of the Eritrean Pharmaceutical Association. Second Revision. Asmara.

_____. Gazette of Eritrean Laws, Proclamation No. 36/1993, A Proclamation to Control Drugs, Medical Supplies, Cosmetics and Sanitary Items. Asmara.

_____. Proclamation of Eritrean Laws No 86/1996: Establishment of Regional Administrations. Asmara.

Hill, Kenneth, C. Abou Zahr, and Wardlaw, T. 2001. "Estimates of Maternal Mortality for 1995". In Bulletin of the World Health Organization. Geneva.

IMF. 2001. *Eritrea Staff Report*. Washington, D.C.

Lagerstedt, Adam. 2000. *Trip Report on Health Sector Vision and Health Policy Review*. Asmara: Ministry of Health.

Macro International, Inc. 2002. *Eritrea Demographic Health Survey 2002, Preliminary Report*. Maryland.

Management Sciences for Health. 2001. *International Drug Price Indicator Guide*.

_____. 1997. *Managing Drug Supply*.

Ministry of Health. 1997a. *Eritrea: Household Health Status, Utilization and Expenditures Survey*. Asmara.

_____. 1997b. *Eritrean National Drug Policy*, State of Eritrea. Final Draft. Asmara.

_____. 1998. *Eritrean Standard Treatment Guidelines*. Asmara.

_____. 1999. *Eritrea Health Laboratory Survey, 1998/99*. Central Health Laboratory.

_____. 2000a. *Annual Health Service Activity Report (January–December 1999)*. Asmara.

_____. 2000b. *Concept Paper for the Health Sector Review*. Asmara.

_____. 2000c. *Health Management Information Systems Report*. Asmara.

_____. 2001a. *Annual Health Service Activity Report (January–December 2000)*. Asmara.

_____. 2001b. *Eritrea Health Profile 2000: EPI Coverage Survey*. Asmara.

_____. 2001c. *Eritrean National List of Drugs*. 3rd Edition. Asmara.

_____. 2001d. *Health profile 2000*. Asmara.

_____. 2002. Finance Office. *Sources and Uses of Revenues for the Health Sector, 1999 and 2002*. Asmara.

Sebhatu, M. *et.al.* 1994. "Eritrea, Summary Report". In *Proceedings of the East Africa Burden of Disease, Cost-Effectiveness of Health Care Interventions and Health Policy*. pp. 33–42. Regional Workshop. August 17–19, 1994. Asmara.

Tekeste, Assefaw, G. Tsehaye, and M. Dagnew. 1999. *Health Needs Assessment of the Eritrean Nomadic Communities*. Asmara: Ministry of Health and University of Asmara.

Tseggai, A. 1998. "Human Resource Development: Priorities for Policy". In *Post Conflict Eritrea: Prospects for Reconstruction and Development*, ed. *by* Doombos, Martin and A. Tesfai. New Jersey: Red Sea Press.

UNAIDS/WHO. 2001. *Epidemiological Fact Sheet for Eritrea on HIV/AIDS and Sexually Transmitted Infection*. 2000 Update, (online) UNAIDS Website. Geneva.

UNFPA. 2000. *The State of World Population*, (online) UNICEF Website. New York.

UNICEF. 2001a. *Global Database on Antenatal Care*, (online) UNICEF Website. New York.

_____. 2001b. *Global Database on Births Attended by Skilled Health Personnel*, (online) UNICEF Website. New York

WHO. 1993. *How to Investigate Drug Use in Health Facilities, Action Programme on Essential Drugs*. Geneva.

_____. 1994. *Indicators for Monitoring National Drug Policies, Action Programme on Essential Drugs*. Geneva.

_____. 2000a. Global Database on Child Growth and Malnutrition, (online) WHO Website.

_____. 2000b. *Global Summary, Department of Vaccines and Biological* (online) WHO Website. Geneva.

_____. 2000c. *The Use of Essential Drugs*. Ninth Report of the WHO Expert Committee. Geneva.

_____. 2000d. *Vaccine Preventable Diseases: Monitoring System*. Geneva.

_____. 2000e. *World Health Report 2000. Health Systems: Improving Performance*. Geneva.

World Bank. 1997. *Project Appraisal Document for Eritrea Health Project*. Human Development IV/Africa Region (Report No. 16501-ER). Washington, D.C.: World Bank.

_____. 2001. *World Development Indicators*. Washington, D.C.

_____. 2002. *Eritrea – Health Sector Note*. Washington, D.C.

Yoder, R. 1995. "Health Facilities Cost Estimates Study." In *Eritrean Health and Population Project*, BASICS Project.

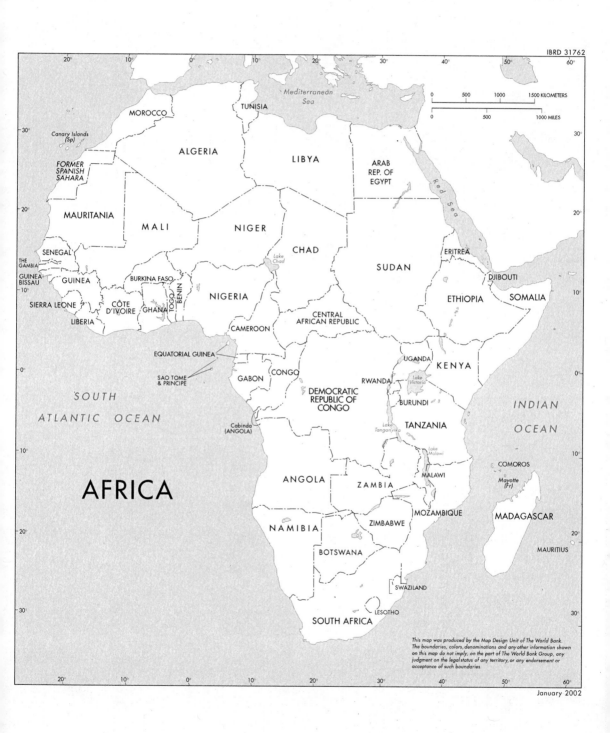

IBRD 31762

Mediterranean Sea

MOROCCO

TUNISIA

Canary Islands (Sp)

FORMER SPANISH SAHARA

ALGERIA

LIBYA

ARAB REP. OF EGYPT

Red Sea

MAURITANIA

MALI

NIGER

CHAD

SUDAN

ERITREA

DJIBOUTI

SENEGAL

THE GAMBIA

GUINEA-BISSAU

GUINEA

BURKINA FASO

Lake Chad

NIGERIA

ETHIOPIA

SOMALIA

SIERRA LEONE

CÔTE D'IVOIRE

GHANA

TOGO

BENIN

LIBERIA

CAMEROON

CENTRAL AFRICAN REPUBLIC

EQUATORIAL GUINEA

SAO TOME & PRINCIPE

GABON

CONGO

UGANDA

KENYA

RWANDA

Lake Victoria

DEMOCRATIC REPUBLIC OF CONGO

BURUNDI

SOUTH

ATLANTIC OCEAN

Cabinda (ANGOLA)

Lake Tanganyika

TANZANIA

INDIAN

OCEAN

Lake Malawi

COMOROS

AFRICA

ANGOLA

ZAMBIA

MALAWI

Mayotte (Fr)

MOZAMBIQUE

MADAGASCAR

NAMIBIA

ZIMBABWE

MAURITIUS

BOTSWANA

SWAZILAND

LESOTHO

SOUTH AFRICA

This map was produced by the Map Design Unit of The World Bank. The boundaries, colors, denominations and any other information shown on this map do not imply, on the part of The World Bank Group, any judgment on the legal status of any territory, or any endorsement or acceptance of such boundaries.

0 500 1000 1500 KILOMETERS

0 500 1000 MILES

January 2002